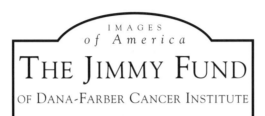

IMAGES
of America

THE JIMMY FUND
OF DANA-FARBER CANCER INSTITUTE

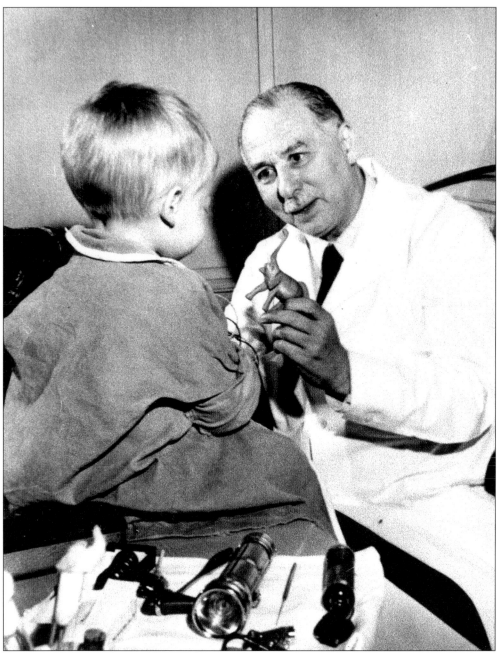

DR. SIDNEY FARBER AT WORK, 1966. As founder of the Children's Cancer Research Foundation (now Dana-Farber Cancer Institute), Dr. Sidney Farber used his talents as a world-renowned researcher and a warm-hearted clinician to ensure that patients received the best possible care. He was determined to improve the often grim recovery rates for childhood diseases and to bring about a revolution in how both young and adult patients were treated. "I have never accepted the incurability of cancer," Farber once stated. "And I have remained hopeful, not because of wishful thinking—that's not progress—but because of the factual evidence of progress. There is no such thing as a hopeless case." (Jimmy Fund.)

IMAGES
of America

THE JIMMY FUND

OF DANA-FARBER CANCER INSTITUTE

Saul Wisnia

To Vickie + Vanessa Roldan—
Whose beautiful faces grace
the last page of this book.
Thank you for all your
support of Dana-Farber,

ARCADIA

First printed in 2002.

Published by Arcadia Publishing,
an imprint of Tempus Publishing, Inc.
2A Cumberland Street
Charleston, SC 29401

Printed in Great Britain.

Library of Congress Catalog Card Number: 2002106081

For all general information contact Arcadia Publishing at:
Telephone 843-853-2070
Fax 843-853-0044
E-Mail sales@arcadiapublishing.com

For customer service and orders:
Toll-Free 1-888-313-2665
Visit us on the internet at http://www.arcadiapublishing.com

All Steve Gilbert photographs copyrighted 1984–2002.

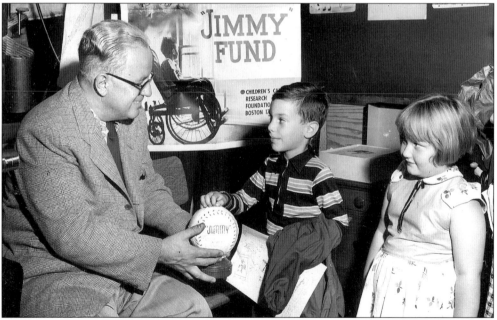

"BIG BROTHER" BOB EMERY COLLECTS FOR JIMMY, C. THE 1950S. One of the most ardent supporters of the Jimmy Fund during the charity's early years was veteran Boston radio and television personality Bob Emery (left). His popular children's television show *Big Brother's Small Fry Club* featured a combination of celebrity interviews, cartoons, and educational tips. When not at his studio, Emery could often be found at Children's Hospital, singing and entertaining patients. During one Jimmy Fund appeal, he had Dr. Sidney Farber appear on his program and mailed collection kits to his young viewers, a combination that generated $11,000. (Jimmy Fund.)

CONTENTS

ACKNOWLEDGMENTS

The writing of this book took place in early 2002, but my connection to the Jimmy Fund goes back much further. As a young boy growing up in Newton, Massachusetts, I was keenly aware of the charity and the special place it held in the hearts of many New Englanders. I saw the familiar billboard in right field on visits to Fenway Park and heard Ken Coleman pitch numerous Jimmy Fund promotions while I listened to Red Sox games on the radio. As a Little Leaguer in the mid-1970s, I went door-to-door for the cause in my sweltering wool uniform. While researching this project, I was amused to learn that David Perini Sr., son of the Boston Braves owner who helped found the Jimmy Fund, had done the same three decades before.

For many years after this, my only real connection to the Jimmy Fund was supporting friends in their various runs, walks, and other endeavors for the charity. Then, three years ago, I found myself back in the fold, this time as a publications editor and writer at Dana-Farber Cancer Institute (DFCI). Suddenly I was faced day-to-day with the real stories behind the events: the brave patients and committed staff who make Dana-Farber and the Jimmy Fund so special. Already aware of the wonderful tale behind the charity's formation, I was able to meet and befriend Einar "Jimmy" Gustafson himself and was even one of Ted Williams' tour guides on his dramatic return to the institute. I also became a dedicated participant in numerous Jimmy Fund events and was moved by the determination of patients young and old walking or running alongside me.

The idea to take all these powerful moments and put them into a book came from my longtime friend and mentor, Richard Johnson. Author of Arcadia Publishing's volume on the Boston Braves, he encouraged me to take on this project—which turned into a labor of love supported by many people. First and foremost are my colleagues on the communications staff at Dana-Farber. All assisted in one way or another, but several deserve special mention. My bosses Paul Hennessy and Steven Singer backed the project from the start. The superb science writing of Robert Levy—particularly his stories on the early years of Dana-Farber and the Jimmy Fund—was immensely helpful. Alessandra Ciambra, John DiGianni, Kristin Lacey, Karalyn Leavens, Kimberly Regensburg, and Caroline Woodcheke aided in my photograph searches and scanning requests. Karen Cummings and Debbie Ruder provided more support than either will ever know—editing, sharing stories, picking out photographs (including their own), and just being there as friends. Any success this project enjoys is due in great part to their efforts.

The photographers past and present whose stellar work enlivens the pages that follow are also in my debt. Steve Gilbert and Mark Ostow, in particular, were generous with their time and images, but my thanks also go to any others whose shots appear here, as well as to John Cronin and Hank Hryniewicz of the Boston Herald, the Brearley Collection, the New England Sports Museum, and Ralph Edwards Productions. Dr. George Foley's internally published account of Dana-Farber's first 25 years, The House That Jimmy Built, was a great source for information, as were old Dana-Farber publications such as Centerline. Mort Lederman, whose career at Dana-Farber spans 50 years, furnished key names and photographs. Bill Nowlin's research was of vital assistance, as were stories shared by Drs. David Nathan, Emil Frei III, and other Dana-Farber leaders. Mike Andrews, Suzanne Fountain, and Jenny Cooper of the Jimmy Fund came through when I needed them.

Lastly, I thank my wife, Michelle, and son, Jason, for their love, support, and for putting up with the lonely nights and crazy days as I lost myself in photographs and captions. Jason's first words were "Daddy, bye" as he saw me go off on yet another archival excursion; I was hoping for "Red Sox," but I guess this will make a better story.

INTRODUCTION

"I have had a chance to see for myself some of the sick children who are suffering from cancer, as well as the wonderful work being done by this great and kind man, Dr. Sidney Farber, and that staff in the Jimmy Fund Building.

"The way I look at it, there is always something we can do for some youngster somewhere. Here, we don't have to look any further than the Jimmy Fund. Somehow, it strikes me that a dollar tossed into this drive is the whole American way of life in a nutshell. All the bullets and all the bombs that explode all over the world won't leave the impact, when all is said or done, of a dollar bill dropped in the Jimmy Fund pot by a warm heart and a willing hand. . . . You should be proud and happy to know that your contribution will someday help some kid to a better life."

—Ted Williams, August 17, 1953, at a welcome-home dinner held to benefit the Jimmy Fund after his return from the Korean War. For a half-century of devotion to the charity, Williams was later named an honorary trustee for life of Dana-Farber Cancer Institute.

When Dr. Sidney Farber was toiling away in a small basement laboratory in Boston's Children's Hospital shortly after World War II, childhood cancer was almost universally fatal. Today, the recovery rate for some forms of the disease is as high as 90 percent, thanks in large part to the chemotherapy treatments developed by Farber in those early days. His modest one-room facility of the late 1940s has transformed into Dana-Farber Cancer Institute (DFCI), where roughly 3,000 physicians, nurses, researchers, and support staff continue seeking cures for pediatric and adult cancers, AIDS, and related diseases while providing the best possible care to today's patients and their families.

The remarkable story of the charity that helped this center grow from Farber's dream to a world-renowned institution unfolds on the following pages. Starting with a 1948 radio broadcast from the hospital bedside of one of Farber's young patients known only as Jimmy, the fund quickly became a New England phenomenon. Over the past five-plus decades, countless individuals and groups have contributed through cash donations or by walking, biking, golfing, and more in the charity's many fundraisers. From the first coins collected after that original radio show, the Jimmy Fund has generated more than $200 million for Dana-Farber. Today, there are more than 300 events held annually, with an average of 85¢ per dollar raised going directly toward DFCI's ultimate goal of eradicating cancer and related diseases.

In addition to becoming recognized as "New England's favorite charity," the Jimmy Fund has partnered with other beloved regional institutions. The Jimmy Fund is the official cause of the Boston Red Sox, and its long history with baseball extends back to the fund's formation. The Jimmy Fund, however, involves more than America's pastime. It is also the official charity of the Massachusetts Chiefs of Police Association, the Variety Club of New England, and the Pan-Massachusetts Challenge bike-a-thon (the largest bicycling fundraiser in the country). Each summer, more than 200 cinemas from Maine to Florida raise money for Dana-Farber through the Jimmy Fund/Variety Club Theatre Collections Program, as ushers pass around Jimmy Fund canisters for patrons to plunk in their coins or bills. The tradition has endured in movie houses and drive-ins since 1949 and brings in more than $1.5 million annually.

Where does all the money go? It helps the institute's numerous programs probing the causes of cancer—a group of diseases expected to kill more than half a million people in the United States during 2002, or more than 1,500 people per day. Funds also go toward providing care for the thousands of pediatric and adult patients who walk through Dana-Farber's doors each year and toward supporting their families.

Among the beneficiaries is Andrew MacKinlay, a nine-year-old Massachusetts boy treated for acute lymphoblastic leukemia in the Jimmy Fund Clinic and at Children's Hospital in Boston. Thanks to the care he has received, MacKinlay can dream the same dreams as other youngsters. "I really want to go to college and play basketball like my dad," he said in a speech given to Dana-Farber friends in 2001. "One day maybe I will tell my college basketball teammates that I had leukemia, and that it was the hardest thing I have ever done. Maybe then chemo will be easier for kids, and they won't have to feel sick for so long. I like to think about that."

Those moved by seeing this young man and patients of all ages go forward with their lives include Jimmy Fund chairman Mike Andrews, a former Red Sox infielder who has worked on staff with the charity for the past 23 years.

"I was able to play in two World Series, and win one of them," Andrews recalls. "I played in an All-Star game and had 13 wonderful years in professional baseball. I loved the game, but it gave me nowhere near the satisfaction that I've enjoyed being part of Dana-Farber's mission to help cure these dreaded diseases.

"To watch the Jimmy Fund grow as it has—along with the cure rates for cancer—is fantastic. It's a critical part of Dana-Farber's success, and it's great to be doing something so worthwhile."

This book is dedicated to Dr. Sidney Farber, to Einar "Jimmy" Gustafson, and to all the patients treated at Dana-Farber Cancer Institute and helped by the Jimmy Fund since 1948.

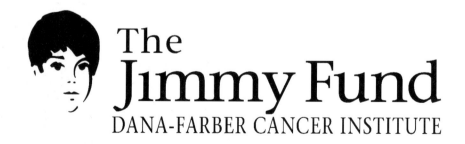

One

A Man Named Farber, a Boy Named Jimmy: The Beginning

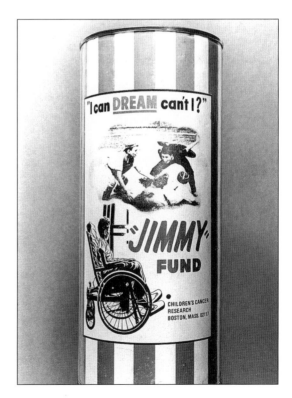

A Jimmy Fund Collection Canister, c. 1950. After the moving radio appearance in May 1948 by an anonymous 12-year-old cancer patient at Boston's Children's Hospital, "Jimmy" was soon a household name throughout New England. Jimmy Fund collection canisters like this one could be found wherever appeals to support the work of Dr. Sidney Farber and the Children's Cancer Research Foundation were held in the six-state region. (Jimmy Fund.)

The tale of the Jimmy Fund starts with two individuals—a fiercely determined doctor and a sick little boy.

The third oldest of 14 siblings, Sidney Farber was born in Buffalo, New York, in 1903 and graduated from the University of Buffalo at age 20. After a year studying medicine in Germany, he settled in Boston and completed Harvard Medical School with the Class of 1927. Although he would make landmark cancer discoveries with worldwide implications over the following decades, his home office would almost always remain within a few blocks of the Harvard Medical School campus.

Farber did his graduate training in pathology at Peter Bent Brigham Hospital (now Brigham and Women's Hospital) and, in 1928, was appointed a resident pathologist at Children's Hospital and an assistant in pathology at Harvard Medical School. A year later, he was named the hospital's first full-time pathologist and quickly developed a reputation as a top scientist and vibrant lecturer. Frustrated by the often hopeless prognosis for pediatric cancer patients, he helped in 1946 to create the Children's Medical Center, a consortium of seven institutions including Children's Hospital. The next year, he became the center's pathologist-in-chief.

In the period after World War II, Farber focused his research on leukemia. Since it was first identified in 1845, the disease had remained 100 percent fatal for children and adults, and patients usually died within weeks of diagnosis. Driven to change these grim results, Farber labored in a single microbiology laboratory room in the basement of Children's Hospital. He was aided, as the story goes, "by one assistant and 10,000 mice."

Leukemia is a disease of the white blood cell–making tissue of the bone marrow, and Farber's theory for halting its progression involved chemically blocking the folic acid that stimulated the growth and maturation of bone marrow. Using a drug called Aminopetrin for this purpose on 16 young leukemia patients in November 1947, he achieved temporary remissions (including the disappearance of tumors) in 10 of them.

When reported in the June 3, 1948 issue of the *New England Journal of Medicine,* these findings were initially met with skepticism by many in the scientific community, since no drug had ever been proven effective against non-solid tumors (those that are spread throughout the body and cannot be surgically removed). Physicians who were intrigued enough to contact Farber about their patients received personal responses, and the one-room tumor clinic in Children's Hospital was soon moved to a larger site in a nearby apartment building.

During this period, in a case of perfect timing, Farber met the man who would become his longtime professional partner—William S. "Bill" Koster. In 1947, Koster was executive director of the Variety Club of New England, a social and giving organization connected with the theater and entertainment industry. Made wealthy by the World War II movie-making boom, club members were looking for charitable causes to support. They were already backing the blood bank at Children's Hospital when they came upon Farber's basement laboratory during a tour of the facility. Koster was immediately intrigued by the dynamic physician and his dream.

Under Koster's leadership, the Variety Club held a theater raffle throughout New England to establish the Children's Cancer Research Foundation (CCRF) and bolster Farber's work. A March 1948 fundraising drive netted $45,536 for the foundation, and then came an even more ambitious appeal: a live radio broadcast from the bedside of one of the doctor's young patients.

Thanks largely to George Swartz, a Variety Club member in Boston with Hollywood connections, the event would be aired nationally by host Ralph Edwards on his popular show *Truth or Consequences.* The child chosen by Farber to chat with Edwards was 12-year-old Einar Gustafson, a friendly youngster from the tiny town of New Sweden, Maine, near the Canadian border. The tall, blond farmer's son was being treated for Burkitt's non-Hodgkin's lymphoma, a form of cancer then fatal in about 85 percent of pediatric patients. He also happened to be a fan of the Boston Braves, the city's National League baseball club. When this news reached Braves publicist Billy Sullivan, he convinced team owner Louis Perini to back the project as well.

The Saturday night broadcast started with Edwards speaking before a live studio audience in Hollywood and then cut to the Children's Hospital room of Gustafson, identified only as

"Jimmy" to protect his privacy. As the two chatted coast-to-coast, Braves players appeared in the room on cue with autographed balls, bats, and jerseys for Gustafson. Manager Billy Southworth entered last with an authentic woolen team uniform tailored to the boy's size and a promise of one victory in the next day's doubleheader if he came out to watch.

Once the group had assembled by Gustafson's bed, a piano was rolled in and Jimmy led a rendition of "Take Me Out to the Ballgame." His excited, off-key voice could be heard above the rest. After the radio feed from Boston ended, Edwards concluded the broadcast with an appeal that if listeners donated $20,000 to the Children's Cancer Research Fund, Jimmy would get a television set to view his beloved Braves in action. When Edwards suggested to Farber that his foundation's name was too long for people to remember, the researcher-turned-fundraiser quickly offered an alternative for solicitation purposes—the Jimmy Fund.

The response was immediate. Nearby listeners walked or drove to Children's Hospital with cash donations minutes after Edwards went off the air, and telegrams and letters bearing additional contributions flooded in from across the country. Gustafson went to Braves Field the next day to see his new friends beat the Cubs twice, and within a week, Braves players had purchased their own $1,000 television and had given it to Jimmy. For the rest of the summer, these big-leaguers used what free time they had in the heat of a pennant race to appear at fundraisers statewide for their team's new official charity. Thousands of other individuals and organizations from cities and towns across New England followed suit with bake sales, concerts, parades, and other efforts. Louis Perini's son, Dana-Farber trustee David Perini Sr., remembers doing his part by going door-to-door in his Little League uniform on sweltering summer nights for donations. By autumn, these combined efforts resulted in a phenomenal $231,485.51 raised for Farber and the Children's Cancer Research Foundation.

Einar Gustafson returned to Maine that same fall to start his long recovery, but the Jimmy Fund was in Boston to stay. The charity's now familiar collection canisters began making their way through the aisles at movie theaters and drive-ins the next summer, and ground was broken in late 1949 on the five-story Jimmy Fund Building to replace Farber's one-room laboratory. When it opened just over two years later, the structure fulfilled the researcher's dream of a center dedicated entirely to the research and treatment of childhood cancers. It was the first such facility of its kind in the country.

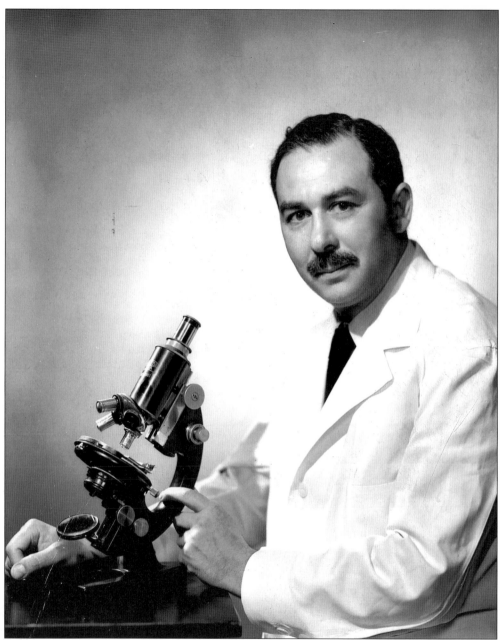

DR. SIDNEY FARBER, C. 1947. Dr. Sidney Farber was driven throughout his medical career by a single, powerful idea. He was convinced that the only thing standing between cancer science and cures was forceful, diligent research, sufficient funding, and the national will to bring it about. While still a young pathologist at Children's Hospital in Boston, he achieved the first clinical remission with chemotherapy ever reported for childhood leukemia—earning him status as "the father of modern chemotherapy." He then spent nearly 30 years improving on his startling results, launching one of the world's premier cancer centers along the way.

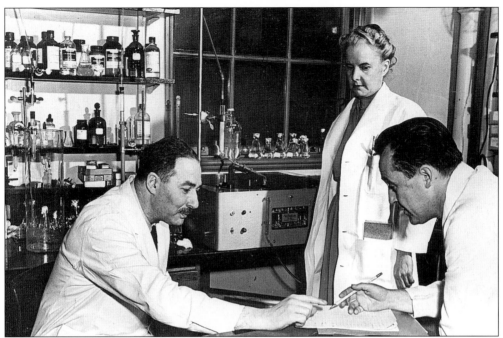

MODEST QUARTERS, C. 1950. Shown here with colleagues Drs. Virginia Downing and George E. Foley, Farber (left) spent the years following World War II conducting his breakthrough cancer research in a 9- by 12-foot microbiology laboratory housed in the basement of the Department of Pathology at Children's Hospital. (Jimmy Fund.)

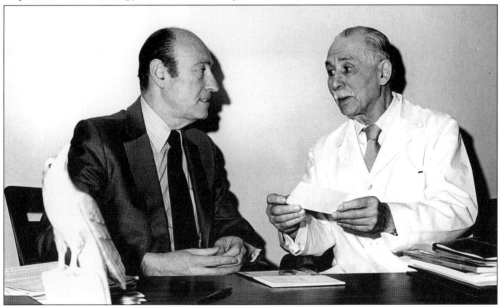

BILL KOSTER AND SIDNEY FARBER, PARTNERS. From the moment they met in 1947, Sidney Farber (right) and Bill Koster from the Variety Club of New England formed a truly dynamic duo. They developed the Children's Cancer Research Foundation into a powerful entity through Farber's brilliant medical skills and Koster's ability to go anywhere and do anything if it yielded a check for the Jimmy Fund. Their partnership lasted more than 25 years. (Jimmy Fund.)

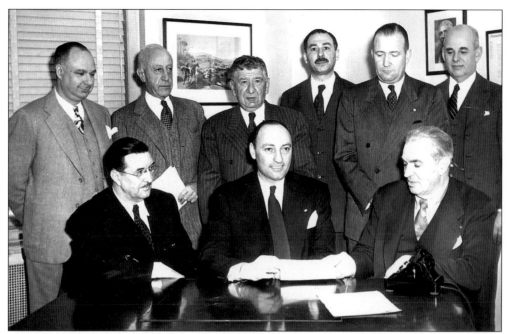

THE VARIETY CLUB COMPLETES THE FIRST CCRF DRIVE, MARCH 1948. In its initial campaign for the Children's Cancer Research Foundation (CCRF), the Variety Club collected $45,536 during the winter of 1948. In this view, Bill Koster (front, center) presents a check to CCRF treasurer Murray Weiss (left) and president John Dervin while other club members and Sidney Farber look on. (Jimmy Fund.)

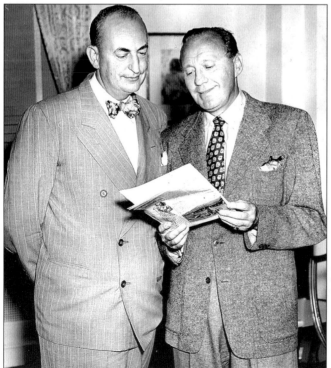

GEORGE SWARTZ AND JACK BENNY, 1948. A prominent Boston insurance agent and Variety Club member, George Swartz (left) had Hollywood connections that included radio stars Jack Benny, Eddie Cantor, and Ralph Edwards. With their help, he had raised more than $1 million for the Infantile Paralysis Fund; now he sought their assistance to promote the work of Farber and the CCRF with a national radio appeal for the foundation. (Jimmy Fund.)

RALPH EDWARDS, THE LATE 1940s. Host of the top-rated *Truth or Consequences* audience-participation radio show, Ralph Edwards already had commitments to other charitable efforts when Swartz approached him about focusing a show around Farber. "There are no prior rights over sick children," Swartz told him. "This is not just a Boston thing. This is something that reaches every youngster all over the world." Convinced, Edwards made arrangements for the broadcast. (Ralph Edwards Productions.)

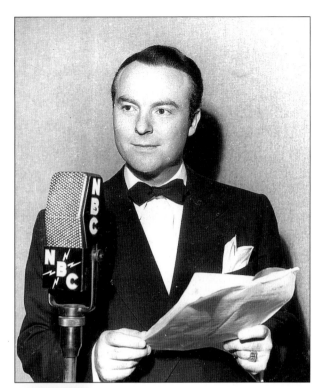

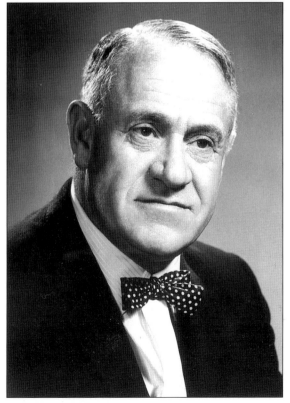

LOUIS PERINI, C. 1948. Owner with his brothers of a construction business and a portion of the Boston Braves baseball club, Perini had helped make both entities a huge success. As president of the Braves, he had the club in contention for a National League championship by 1948, when team publicist Billy Sullivan first told him about Farber's efforts to eradicate children's cancer. Like Edwards, Perini was moved to help, setting the stage for the dramatic events that followed. (Jimmy Fund.)

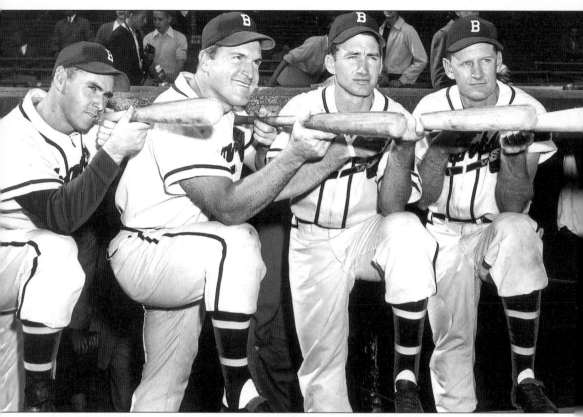

THE BOSTON BRAVES GO TO BAT FOR JIMMY, MAY 1948. The Braves were at the height of their popularity in 1948. The team featured standout hitters—including, from left to right, Tommy Holmes, Jeff Heath, Al Dark, and Bob Elliott—along with baseball's best pitching duo in John Sain and Warren Spahn. Among the team's ardent fans was Einar Gustafson, a 12-year-old cancer patient being treated at Children's Hospital by Dr. Sidney Farber. In May 1948, George Swartz of the Variety Club, working with Braves owner Lou Perini and team publicist Billy Sullivan, arranged for the boy to meet his baseball heroes in his hospital room while a nationwide radio audience listened on the Ralph Edwards *Truth or Consequences* program. Dubbed "Jimmy" to guard his privacy, the youngster won the hearts of the players and millions more during the eight-minute broadcast. When Braves broadcaster Jim Britt recounted details of the performance to his listeners the next day, the message spread even further. (Boston Herald.)

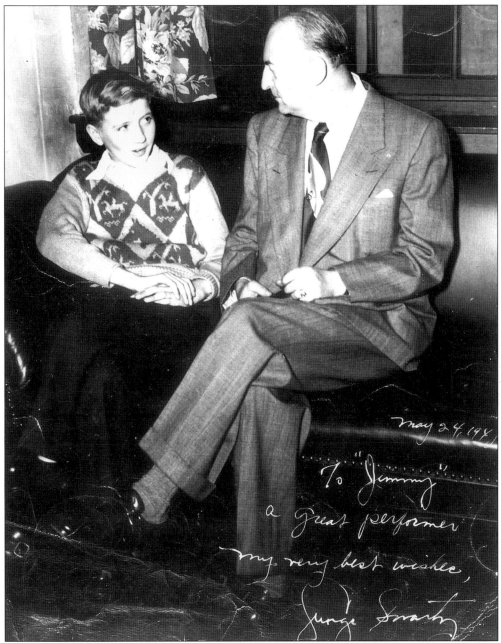

Einar "Jimmy" Gustafson and George Swartz after the Show, May 24, 1948. Although the Jimmy broadcast had been hyped beforehand in Boston newspapers, no one foresaw the dramatic impact it had on those who heard it. Einar Gustafson displayed a genuine enthusiasm that prompted an outpouring of support for the boy and the Children's Cancer Research Foundation. People walking or driving by Children's Hospital headed to the front desk with change and dollar bills, and telegraphic money orders arrived from as far away as California the same night. Here, Gustafson and George Swartz of the Variety Club, who arranged the show, relax two days after making history. The inscription from Swartz reads, "To 'Jimmy'—a great performer." (Gustafson family collection.)

The following are excerpts from the eight-minute radio broadcast that launched the Jimmy Fund. Host Ralph Edwards performed on May 22, 1948, in front of a live Hollywood audience and talked to his guests in Boston by remote hook-up.

RALPH EDWARDS: Part of the function of *Truth or Consequences* is to bring this old parlor game to people who are unable to come to the show, and tonight we take you to a little fellow named Jimmy. We're not going to give you his last name, because he's just like thousands of other young fellows and girls in private homes and hospitals all over the country. Jimmy is suffering from cancer. He's a swell little guy, and although he can't figure out why he isn't out with the other kids, he does love his baseball, and follows every move of his favorite team, the Boston Braves.

Now, by the magic of radio, we're going to span the breadth of the United States and take you right up to the bedside of Jimmy in one of America's great cities, Boston, Massachusetts, and into one of America's great hospitals, the Children's Hospital in Boston, whose staff is doing such an outstanding job of cancer research for the cause, not only of Boston children, but children in every city in the world.

Up until now, Jimmy has not heard us. Now, we tune in a speaker in his room in the hospital. All right, engineers—here, and in Boston—give us Jimmy please. Hello, Jimmy?

JIMMY: Hi!

EDWARDS: Hi, Jimmy! This is Ralph Edwards of the *Truth or Consequences* radio program. I've heard you like baseball, is that right?

JIMMY: Yeah, it's my favorite sport!

EDWARDS: Who do you think is going to win the pennant this year?

JIMMY: The Boston Braves, I hope.

EDWARDS: Which one of the Boston Braves is your favorite player?

JIMMY: Johnny Sain.

EDWARDS: Johnny Sain, the pitcher? He's won 20 games two years in a row, hasn't he? And who's the catcher?

JIMMY: Phil Masi.

EDWARDS: That's right, Phil Masi; a member of the National League All-Star team for several seasons. Have you ever met Phil Masi?

JIMMY: No. . . .

MASI: Hi, Jimmy! My name is Phil Masi.

EDWARDS: What? Who is that, Jimmy?!

JIMMY: Phil Masi!

EDWARDS: And where is he?

JIMMY: In my room!

EDWARDS: Well, what do you know?! Right there in your hospital room—Phil Masi from Berlin, Illinois! Who's the best home-run hitter on the team, Jimmy?

JIMMY: Jeff Heath!

HEATH: Thanks, Jimmy! I bet you can sock 'em, too! *(Listeners hear a gasp from Jimmy.)*

EDWARDS: Who's that, Jimmy?

JIMMY: Jeff Heath!

EDWARDS: Wow! Right in your room, there?

JIMMY: Yes!

(As the exchange continues, the group is joined by Braves players Eddie Stanky, Bob Elliott, Earl Torgeson, John Sain, Warren Spahn, Jim Russell, and Tommy Holmes. Each comes with gifts, including T-shirts, autographed photographs, and a game-used bat from Torgeson.)

EDWARDS: Well, there you have it—the first-string Boston Braves baseball team, Jimmy, all in your one room. Is their famous manager Billy Southworth there?

SOUTHWORTH: Yep, I sure am, Ralph! Hello, Jimmy!

JIMMY: Hi!

EDWARDS: There he is, there's Billy Southworth! Everyone is applauding here in Hollywood!

SOUTHWORTH: What do you think of your ballclub, Jimmy?

JIMMY: They're good!

EDWARDS: Jimmy, we saved Billy Southworth for the big surprise at the end. Get a good look at a man who's managed three pennant-winning teams and two World Championship teams. Billy, what's the surprise you've got for young Jimmy, there?

SOUTHWORTH: Well, we play the Chicago Cubs tomorrow in a doubleheader at Braves Field in Boston, and we're calling it "Jimmy's Day." We're dedicating the first game to you, Jimmy. And here's another surprise: a Boston Braves uniform tailored to your size, and a fielder's mitt autographed by yours truly. And dargonit, we're going to win tomorrow's game for you, Jimmy! Aren't we guys?

ALL BRAVES: Yeah!!

EDWARDS: They're going to win it for you tomorrow, Jimmy. It sounds like you're on a winning team. Look, as long as you've got all those baseball men around, how about the bunch of you singing "Take Me Out to the Ballgame?" And Jimmy, you lead us. You know that song, Jimmy?

JIMMY: I think so. . . .

EDWARDS: There's a piano they should be wheeling up to the door of the room now, Jimmy, and a man to play it . . . are you ready, Jimmy?

JIMMY: Yeah!

EDWARDS: Are you ready, Braves?

BRAVES: Yeah! Let's go!

(Everyone sings, with Jimmy in the lead and way off-key; the Hollywood crowd loves it.)

EDWARDS: Jimmy was in there pitching! That was great, Jimmy!

SOUTHWORTH: Harry, if it's OK with the doctors here, we would like to take Jimmy out to the ballgame tomorrow and let him be our guest in a seat right back of home plate!

EDWARDS: Well, where's the director of Children's Hospital? Let's ask him.

DIRECTOR: I'm right here, Ralph, and I think it would do Jimmy a lot of good to get out to Braves Field tomorrow.

EDWARDS: How does that sound, Jimmy?

JIMMY: Great, just swell!

EDWARDS: All right, that's great. Have a good time! So long, Braves, and manager Billy Southworth! I know you fellows want to hang around and talk to Jimmy a few minutes, so we'll get off. So long, Jimmy!!

JIMMY AND BRAVES: Bye!

EDWARDS: So long, and have a swell time at the game, Jimmy! You're a great little guy. Good night, Jimmy!

JIMMY: Thank you very, very much, Mr. Edwards!

EDWARDS: Thank *you* very much, Jimmy, and so long! OK, Johnny—tune out Boston.

(Edwards now gets very subdued, as he was at the beginning of the show.)

Now listen, folks. Jimmy can't hear this, can he? We're not using any photographs of him or using his full name, or he will know about this. Let's make Jimmy and thousands of others boys and girls who are suffering from cancer happy by aiding the research to help find a cure for cancer in children. Because by researching children's cancer, we automatically help the adults and stop it at the outset.

Now, we know one of the things little Jimmy wants most is a television set to watch the baseball games as well as hear them. If you friends would send in your quarters, dollars, and tens of dollars tonight to Jimmy for the Children's Cancer Research Foundation, and over $20,000 or more is contributed for this most worthy cause, we'll see to it that Jimmy gets his television set. Now here's the address for your contribution to Jimmy and the boys and girls of America: Jimmy, Children's Hospital, Boston 15, Massachusetts.

This isn't a contest where you win anything, folks. This is our chance to help little boys and girls like Jimmy win a greater prize: the prize of life.

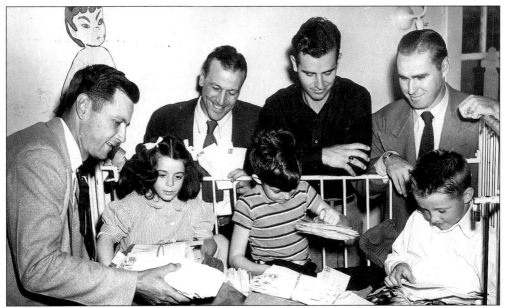

SORTING JIMMY'S FAN MAIL, MAY 1948. In the days following the broadcast, tens of thousands of letters and telegrams from across the country—many in envelopes stuffed with coins and dollar bills, some addressed simply "Jimmy, Boston, Mass."—arrived at Children's Hospital. In this view, Braves players help tackle the deluge with youngsters at the hospital. The players are, from left to right, Johnny Beazley, Phil Masi, an unidentified teammate, and Tommy Holmes. (Jimmy Fund.)

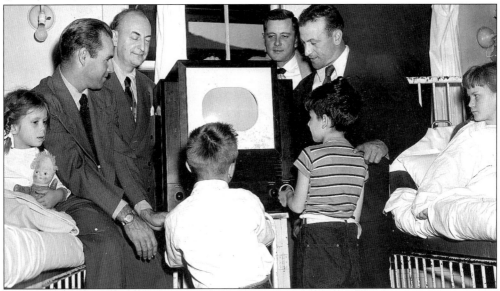

JIMMY GETS HIS TELEVISION, MAY 1948. Just a week after Ralph Edwards promised Jimmy a new television set (then a rare commodity) if listeners could come up with $20,000 in donations, the boy received one—compliments of the Braves team. Players each made personal donations toward the $1,000 set, which was delivered by George Swartz of the Variety Club (at left of set), and players Tommy Holmes, Johnny Beazley, and Phil Masi as Jimmy's pals watched. (Jimmy Fund.)

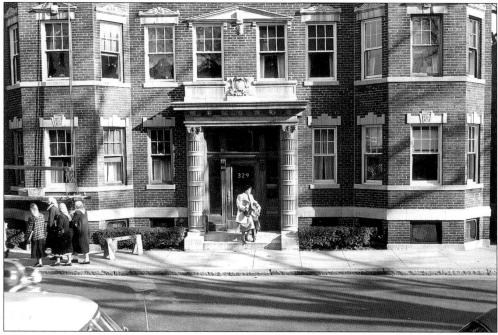

BUZZ HERE FOR THE CHILDREN'S MEDICAL CENTER, C. 1948. While hype from the Jimmy broadcast continued, Dr. Sidney Farber's Aminopetrin research results—in which 10 of 16 leukemia patients went into remission—were reported in the June 3, 1948 issue of the *New England Journal of Medicine*. Soon, patients began arriving for treatment in overwhelming numbers. The outpatient tumor therapy clinic for Children's Medical Center consisted of one room in the Department of Pathology at Children's Hospital, and the onslaught prompted its relocation to bigger quarters in a nearby apartment building (above) on the corner of Longwood Avenue and Binney Street. (Jimmy Fund.)

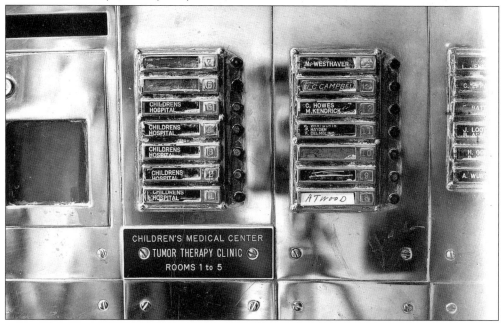

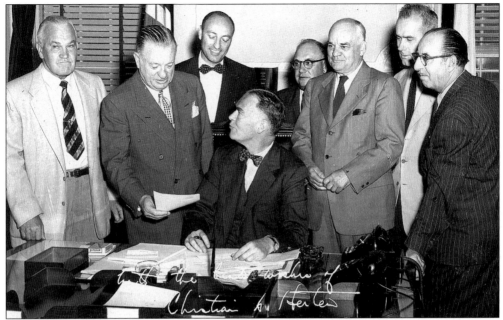

"Jimmy Fund Time" Declared in Massachusetts, Summer 1948. Responding to the outpouring of interest statewide in the new charity, Gov. Christian Herter (seated) officially declared the summer of 1948 Jimmy Fund Time for Massachusetts, as witnessed by a beaming Bill Koster (third from left) and other members of the Variety Club. (Jimmy Fund.)

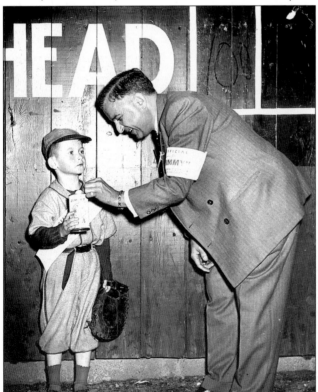

The Jimmy Fund Debut Drive a Huge Success, Summer 1948. By June, "Jimmy Days" were being held throughout New England, with Boston Braves players often in appearance. Thanks to these efforts and the advent of the now familiar Jimmy Fund collection canisters—such as the one Joe Cifre (right) of the Variety Club is adding to here—the campaign brought in an incredible $231,485 by summer's end. (Jimmy Fund.)

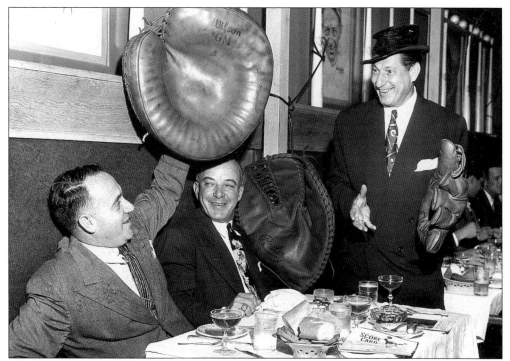

BRAVES GRAB THE PENNANT, SEPTEMBER 1948. Perhaps inspired by their role in launching the Jimmy Fund, the Boston Braves went on to capture their first National League championship in 34 years. At a victory dinner for the team held at Al Schacht's New York restaurant on September 30, Braves owner Lou Perini and manager Billy Southworth celebrated by clowning around with the proprietor. (Boston Herald.)

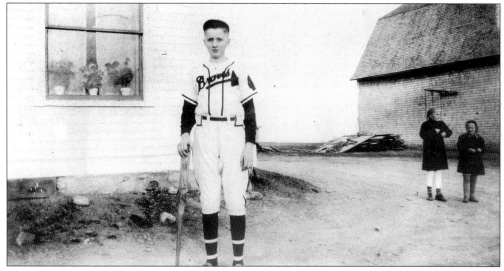

CHERISHED MEMENTOS, C. 1949. In the late 1940s, just 15 percent of children with the type of cancer that Einar "Jimmy" Gustafson had survived the disease. Most people assumed Gustafson was among the casualties, but after his initial treatment in Boston, he returned to Maine and resumed life on his family's potato farm. He poses here with two of his gifts from the Braves—first baseman Earl Torgeson's bat and a regulation team uniform. (Gustafson family collection.)

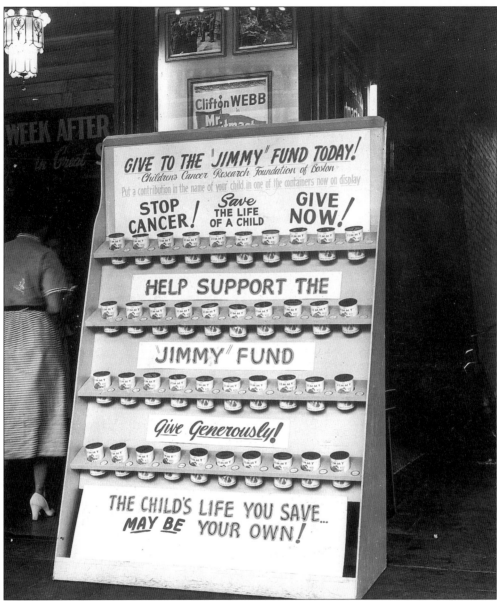

THEATER COLLECTIONS BEGIN, C. 1949. The second Jimmy Fund drive for the Children's Cancer Research Foundation featured the debut of what continues today as the charity's longest-running annual appeal—the Jimmy Fund/Variety Club Theatre Collections Program. During the summer of 1949, displays like this one in Pittsfield, Massachusetts—which featured 40 coin-collection canisters, each emblazoned with the name of a young cancer patient—were placed in lobbies of movie houses and drive-ins throughout the state. Collection canisters were also passed among theater audiences before feature films by ushers and volunteers, including (on some occasions) Boston Red Sox slugger Ted Williams. In the years to come, Williams and Red Sox announcer Curt Gowdy, as well as Hollywood legends Spencer Tracy, Joan Crawford, and Bing Crosby, would make short promotional trailer films about the Jimmy Fund to be shown before canisters were passed around. Today, the program has extended to more than 200 theaters from Maine to Florida and raises more than $1.5 million annually. (Jimmy Fund.)

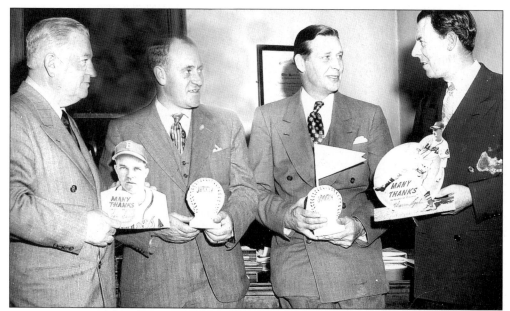

Braves Stars "Pitch" Jimmy Fund Displays, June 1949. The 1949 Jimmy Fund campaign featured cardboard cutouts of Boston Braves players, displayed with the coin-collection canisters. Showing off the models of pennant-winning pitching aces John Sain and Warren Spahn are, from left to right, Martin Mullin (of the Children's Cancer Research Foundation), Lou Perini (Braves owner), Maurice Tobin (U.S. secretary of labor), and John Quinn (Braves general manager). (Boston Herald.)

The Groundbreaking for the Jimmy Fund Building, Fall 1949. After two years of tireless efforts by Bill Koster and the Variety Club, the Jimmy Fund had sufficient funding to begin construction of a state-of-the-art facility for the Children's Cancer Research Foundation. In this view, movie star Burt Lancaster (left) helps Dr. Sidney Farber with "first-digging" honors at the site, which was located at 35 Binney Street in Boston, just a block from Children's Hospital and Harvard Medical School. (Jimmy Fund.)

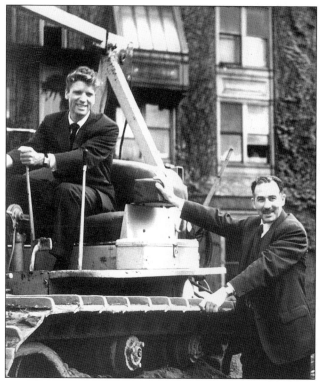

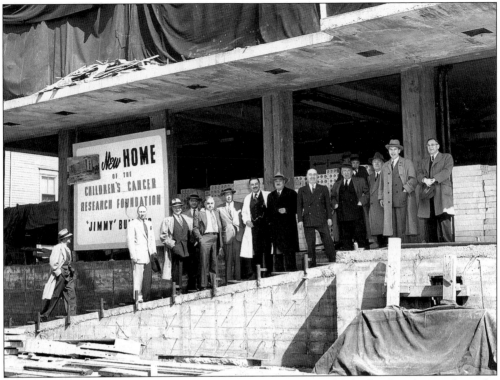

CONSTRUCTION UNDER WAY, 1950. As work continued on the facility known simply as the Jimmy Fund Building, a sharply dressed Sidney Farber (center, with white lab coat) checked out the progress with members of the board of trustees for the Children's Cancer Research Foundation. Bill Koster can be seen at the far left, hat in hand. (Jimmy Fund.)

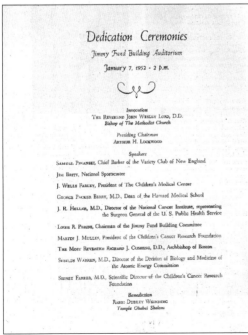

DEDICATION DAY ARRIVES, JANUARY 7, 1952. This page from the booklet given to Jimmy Fund Building dedication attendees shows the key institutions involved with making the structure a reality—medicine, the entertainment industry, and baseball. Following the afternoon ceremony, an evening program was held at Boston's Hotel Statler, featuring speeches by Sidney Farber, Braves owner Lou Perini, and Leonard Goldenson, president of United Paramount Pictures. (Jimmy Fund.)

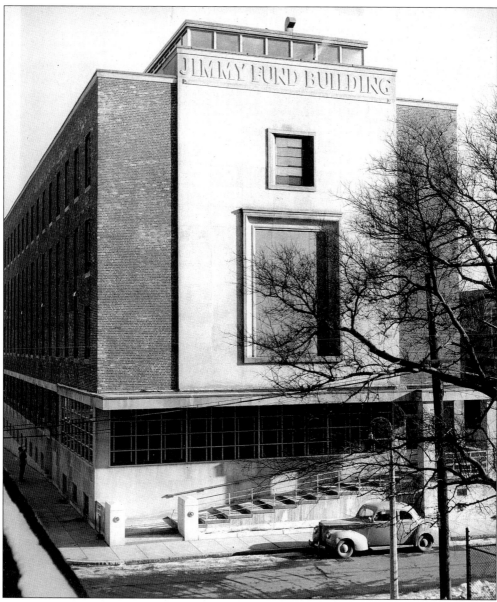

THE JIMMY FUND BUILDING AT ITS COMPLETION, C. 1952. After two-plus years of construction, final costs for "the house that Jimmy built" came to $1.47 million. The Children's Cancer Research Foundation received a $400,000 grant from the National Cancer Institute toward research and laboratory equipment, but most of the expenses were raised by the Jimmy Fund and through private donations. Although all their equipment was not yet in place, many of the 58 Children's Cancer Research Foundation staff members had already moved into the structure by its January dedication ceremonies. The five-story edifice contained generous laboratory and office space in addition to a brand-new outpatient clinic, and staff members were "amazed" by the contrast in size from their previous humble headquarters. Still, Dr. George Foley of the building committee was already looking to the future; he recommended that footings for the building be poured to accommodate the weight of four future floors. It would prove a wise decision. (Jimmy Fund.)

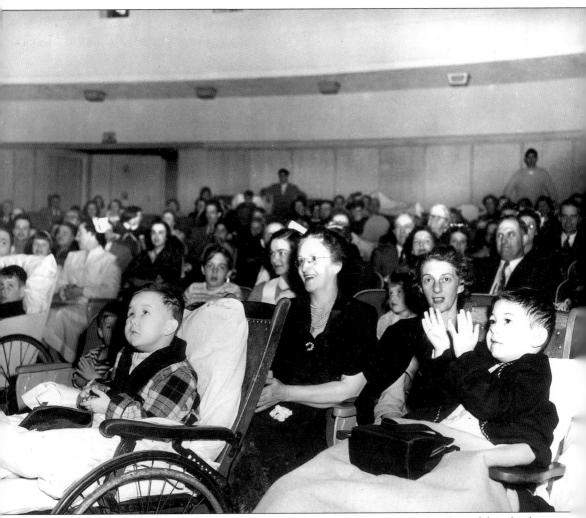

OPENING CEREMONIES ATTRACT KEEN LISTENERS, JANUARY 7, 1952. Seated beside the assorted dignitaries at the building's dedication were the day's most important guests—Sidney Farber's young patients. Among the many tributes written for the occasion were these words from Richard J. Cushing, archbishop of Boston. "I just came from the inaugural ceremony of the new mayor and city government of the City of Boston. I think this is a greater inaugural ceremony," Cushing said. "The former pertained to taxes, the problems of transportation, the assessment of real estate, and other projects identified with the operating of a large metropolitan area. This inaugural pertains to the souls and to the bodies of little children . . . so this is the greater of the two ceremonies that I have attended today." (Jimmy Fund.)

Two

"Teddy Ballgame" and Others Make Their Pitch: 1952–1961

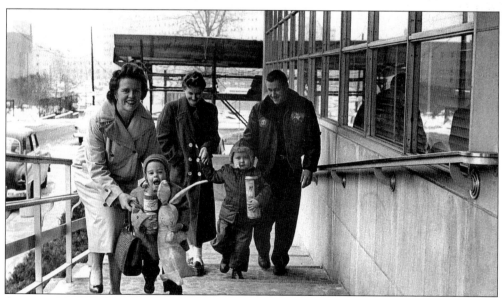

Arriving at the Jimmy Fund Building, c. the 1950s. The first thing patients and families saw when approaching the Jimmy Fund Building were large medallions—one depicting the Variety Club of New England and the other, the Boston Braves—attached to posts on either side of the stairs. The low-rise steps themselves were built wide and at a gradual incline for accommodating little feet and were steam-heated to melt ice and snow. (Jimmy Fund.)

When it opened in January 1952, the Jimmy Fund Building at the Children's Cancer Research Foundation (CCRF) represented a new era in pediatric cancer care. Not only did the five-story structure boast the finest laboratories in the Harvard medical community, but it embodied Dr. Sidney Farber's principles about the care of children with cancer.

The ground floor housed the Jimmy Fund Clinic, where young patients were seen by physicians as well as nutritionists, social workers, and other specialists—a concept that would come to be known as "total patient care." Higher up were state-of-the-art research laboratories, and their proximity to the clinic reflected Farber's belief that scientific advances and clinical care went hand in hand.

Farber "had the idea that if the researchers saw the children as they came in the building, they would be inspired to do better," recalls David G. Nathan, M.D., president of Dana-Farber Cancer Institute (descendant of the CCRF) from 1995 to 2000. "His dream was that on one of the upper floors, a scientist would yell, 'Aha!' and rush down and give a child medicine that would cure him or her." This "bench-to-bedside" philosophy remains true today, both at Dana-Farber and elsewhere. The National Cancer Institute now allocates millions of dollars annually for translational research that aims to convert laboratory discoveries into new therapies.

The Jimmy Fund Building was a short walk but a long way from the tiny laboratory in the basement of Children's Hospital, where Farber had conducted his groundbreaking investigations in previous years. Its construction was the result of more than $1 million collected by the Variety Club of New England through the CCRF's charitable arm, the Jimmy Fund. Help came from varied sources. Countless men, women, and children throughout the region had deposited change into Jimmy Fund canisters at movie theaters and drugstores or had participated in charity events for the cause. More visible supporters from the motion picture industry in Hollywood and the Boston business community had penned checks and hosted functions, and members of the Boston Braves had gone to bat as well.

From parades and billboards to a 10-foot-tall baseball with "pick your favorite player" coin slots, the Jimmy Fund seemed to be everywhere. Coordinating all of the fundraising efforts so that his boss could focus predominantly on research was Bill Koster, the CCRF's executive vice president and Farber's most trusted associate for more than 25 years. Koster read each piece of mail sent to the Jimmy Fund and made sure that every donor, no matter how big or small, received a personal reply. He also devised some outlandish appeals during the fund's infancy, such as the time he persuaded the Prince Macaroni Company and Suffolks Downs Race Track to host "the world's largest spaghetti dinner" for more than 20,000 people. With contributions of $1 per meal (50¢ for children), the pasta-fest was well worth the low overhead needed to run it.

Then, in the early 1950s, a major shake-up in the city's sports scene took place. Ending their 76-year run in Boston, the Braves succumbed to falling attendance and economic woes by departing for Milwaukee in March 1953—leaving the Jimmy Fund without one of its greatest cheerleaders. Braves owner Lou Perini, however, made sure the fund he had helped launch would remain afloat. That spring, he met with Tom Yawkey, the owner of Boston's other major league franchise—the Red Sox—and convinced his colleague to take on the cause as his team's official charity.

Perhaps no single event in Jimmy Fund history was so crucial to its success. Yawkey's decision sparked a relationship that continues a half-century later, making it the longest-known bond between a North American professional sports team and a charity. For many New Englanders, the Red Sox and the Jimmy Fund—located less than a mile apart—have become synonymous.

Yawkey and his wife, Jean, were tremendous supporters of the cause, and no single celebrity has championed the charity's fight against cancer in children and adults more than the Red Sox's all-time greatest star, Ted Williams. From his many unsolicited hospital bed visits to his years as the Jimmy Fund's general chairman and beyond, "the Kid" has used his loyalty, compassion, and towering presence to help stop the disease that claimed the life of his brother Danny and so many others.

Thanks to efforts by Williams, the Yawkeys, the Variety Club, and many others—including the Massachusetts Chiefs of Police Association, which (like the Red Sox) made the fund its official charity in 1953—the Jimmy Fund Building grew to nine stories by decade's end. A suite added for Farber at the top included two offices (one for business, one for patients), a reception area, and even a bed to accommodate his habit of laboring up to 16 hours a day, seven days a week. People still remember looking up at his gleaming office lights late at night and knowing that "Dr. Farber was at work." A second facility, the Jimmy Fund Research Laboratories (later renamed the Michael A. Redstone Laboratories for Animal Research) was added to the campus in 1958.

Although cancer science has changed dramatically since the original building's opening, the structure's life-saving mission has remained unchanged. As J.R. Heller, M.D., then director of the National Cancer Institute, reflected at the 1952 dedication, "This building . . . represents a living, vital, sustaining, very, very great indication of man's humanity to man."

Advances during the early years of the CCRF include the following:

> In 1947, Farber and his team of clinicians and laboratory scientists are the first to attain temporary remissions of acute lymphocytic leukemia (ALL), the most common form of cancer in children. Research that transfers new scientific knowledge "from the lab bench to the bedside" forms the foundation for future progress against cancer at the CCRF (now Dana-Farber Cancer Institute).

> In 1948, Farber's group introduces the first chemotherapy research program in the United States for children with cancer.

> In 1955, the team achieves the first remissions in Wilms' tumor of the kidney, a common form of childhood cancer. Using the antibiotic actinomycin D in addition to surgery and radiation therapy, it boosts cure rates for the disease from 40 percent to 85 percent.

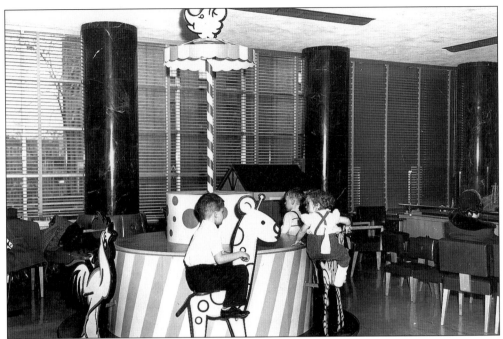

PATIENTS PLAY ON THE CLINIC CAROUSEL, C. 1952. Inside the main waiting room of the Jimmy Fund Clinic was a working carousel for patients and their siblings to ride during their visits. Regularly featured in photographic essays about the Children's Cancer Research Foundation, the merry-go-round remained a treasured part of the clinic for decades to come. (Jimmy Fund.)

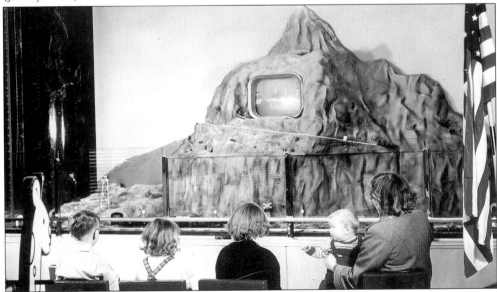

ENJOYING TRAINS AND TELEVISION ON MAGIC MOUNTAIN, C. 1952. Near the carousel was another unique feature of the clinic—Magic Mountain. There, patients and their families could watch television on a screen embedded into a plaster relief of a mountain as they waited for appointments. An electric train that chugged by the television and up the hill provided further entertainment. (Jimmy Fund.)

DISNEY FRIENDS BRIGHTEN THE CLINIC WALLS, C. 1952. One of the most striking characteristics of the new clinic was the examining-room and corridor walls, adorned with 39 colorful oil-based murals featuring Snow White, Pinocchio, Bambi, and other Disney characters in their familiar movie settings. Painted by Dorchester artist Lou Chiarmonte, with permission of Walt Disney Studios, the murals gave patients and caregivers an easy way to tell rooms apart. After the Jimmy Fund Clinic moved to a new building in 1975, the paintings followed five years later. (Jimmy Fund.)

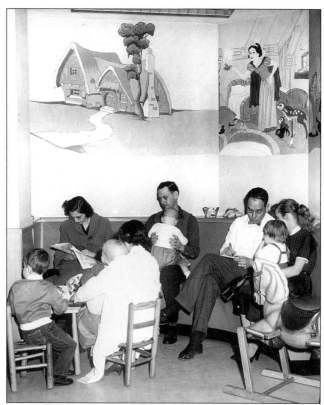

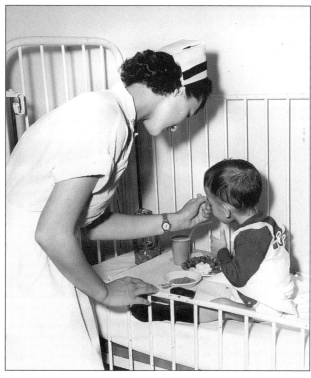

TOTAL PATIENT CARE—THE HALLMARK OF THE CLINIC, C. THE 1950s. Sidney Farber's dream of total patient care was realized with the completion of the Jimmy Fund Building. Patients visiting its inpatient clinic received treatment from physicians and other specialists in a warm, modernized setting, and they had access to additional care as needed from nearby Children's Hospital. (Jimmy Fund.)

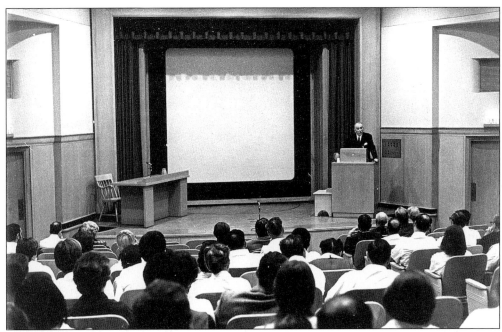

DR. SIDNEY FARBER SPEAKING IN THE JIMMY FUND AUDITORIUM, C. 1969. At its opening in 1952, the 288-seat Jimmy Fund Auditorium was the largest and best-equipped medical amphitheater in Boston. The room's fan shape was expected to cause acoustic problems, but as plans for an elaborate amplification system were being finalized, it was discovered that a coin dropped on the stage could be heard perfectly from every seat in the house. The auditorium is still used today. (Jimmy Fund.)

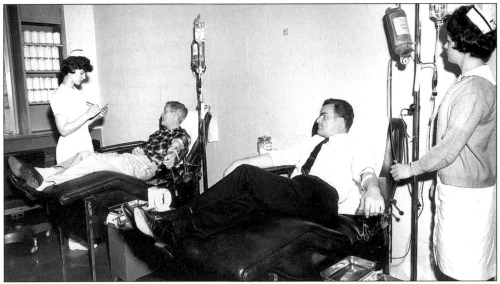

THE BLOOD DONOR CENTER OPENS ITS DOORS, C. THE 1950S. Blood (and later platelet) donors were always welcome at the Jimmy Fund Building, which housed the foundation's donor facility for many years and does so again today, with the opening of the newly refurbished Kraft Family Blood Donor Center there in 2001. The process remains largely the same, but donors now enjoy modern recliners and personal video screens. (Jimmy Fund.)

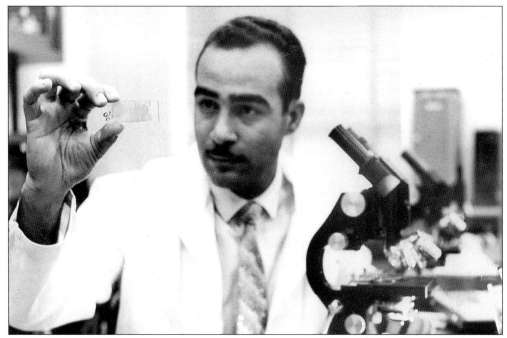

THREE FLOORS FOR RESEARCH, C. THE 1950S. After toiling for years in a one-room basement laboratory, Sidney Farber had three floors of modern research facilities at his disposal in the Jimmy Fund Building. There, a growing team of investigators probed the causes of pediatric cancer while patients received treatment in the building's ground-floor clinic. (Jimmy Fund.)

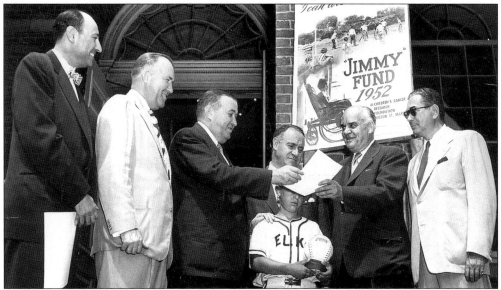

ANOTHER JIMMY FUND DRIVE STARTS, SPRING 1952. With the brand-new Jimmy Fund Building to show for his previous efforts, Bill Koster kicked off his 1952 campaign in style on the steps of the Massachusetts State House. The Little Leaguer standing in front is unidentified. The others are, from left to right, Bill Koster, Massachusetts governor Paul A. Dever, Boston Braves owner Lou Perini, registrar of motor vehicles Rudolph King, and Arthur Lockwood of the Variety Club. (Jimmy Fund.)

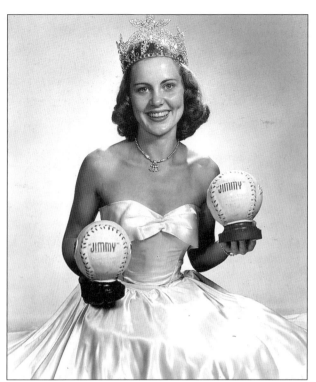

FORMAL-GOWN FUNDRAISING BY MISS MAINE, C. 1952. Norma Lee Collins of Maine did not win the Miss America title in 1952, but she was most likely the best-dressed fundraiser the Jimmy Fund had that year. (Jimmy Fund.)

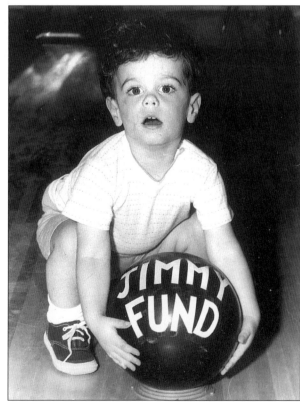

AIMING TO STRIKE OUT CANCER, C. 1953. By the early 1950s, the Jimmy Fund name was clearly embedded in the consciousness of New Englanders, and there was no telling where it might turn up—or roll out—next. (Jimmy Fund.)

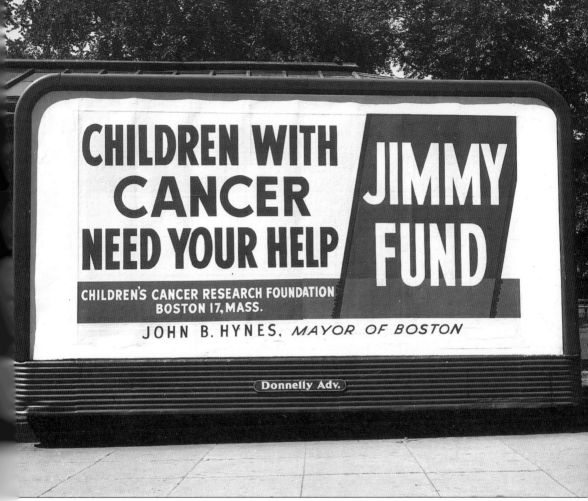

SPREADING THE WORD, C. THE 1950S. Governors in all six New England states declared annual Jimmy Fund Days in the early years of the charity, and support for the popular cause by politicians at all levels has gone on ever since. During the 1950s, Massachusetts governor John B. Hynes used a downtown Boston billboard to get the Children's Cancer Research Foundation message across to passersby. During the 1990s, an analysis of the Jimmy Fund's marketing capabilities determined that the charity maintained a phenomenal 90 percent recognition rate throughout New England. (Jimmy Fund.)

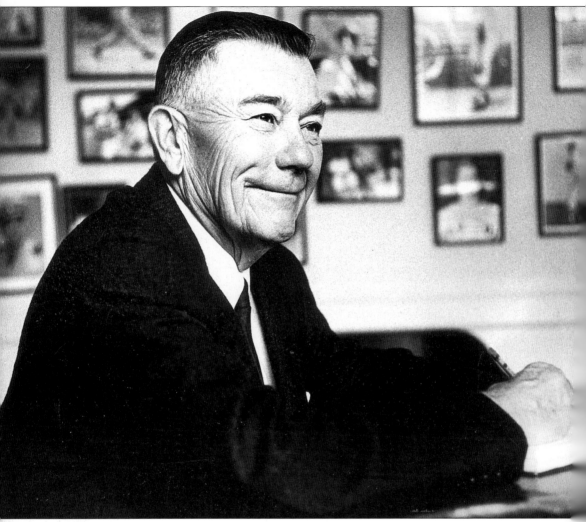

TOM YAWKEY AND THE RED SOX TAKE THE JIMMY FUND REIGNS. When Lou Perini shocked the baseball world by announcing in March 1953 that he was moving the Braves to Milwaukee, he took steps to ensure that the Jimmy Fund–Boston baseball bond would hold by requesting that Red Sox owner Tom Yawkey adopt the cause as his team's official charity. Yawkey complied, and from this point until his death from leukemia in 1976, he and his wife, Jean, were among Sidney Farber's staunchest supporters. Yawkey had banned advertising at Fenway Park around 1950, but soon a Jimmy Fund billboard was erected over the right-field grandstands at the Red Sox's home park—where it remains to this day. Collection boxes were placed throughout Fenway as well, and the Yawkeys made many generous personal contributions. As a tribute to the late couple's benevolence, the Jimmy Fund has established the annual Thomas A. and Jean R. Yawkey Award for dedication to the cause—the highest honor given by the charity. (Jimmy Fund.)

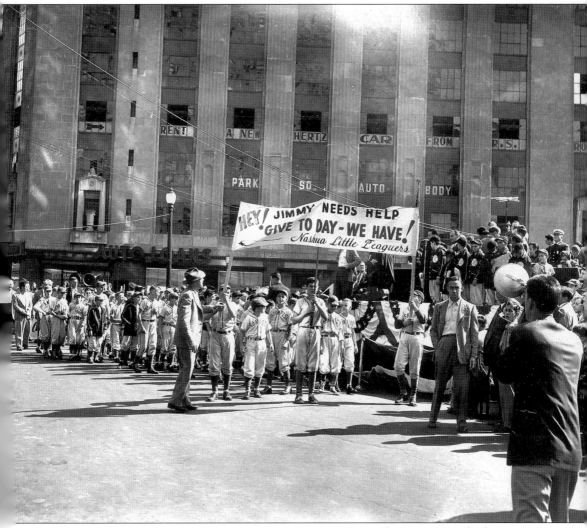

LITTLE LEAGUERS MARCH FOR JIMMY, C. THE 1950S. Since the Jimmy Fund's formation, generations of young baseball players throughout New England (including the author and the contingent shown here) have raised money on Jimmy's behalf by going door-to-door in uniform, hosting bake sales and car washes, and other means. The relationship was made official in 1952 with the formation of the Jimmy Fund Little League Program; each summer since, district baseball and softball teams comprised of players 10 years old and younger have competed on the field and at the collection booth. The top fundraising squads are rewarded with dinner and a Red Sox game at Fenway Park, where they get to see their names in lights on the center-field scoreboard. (Jimmy Fund.)

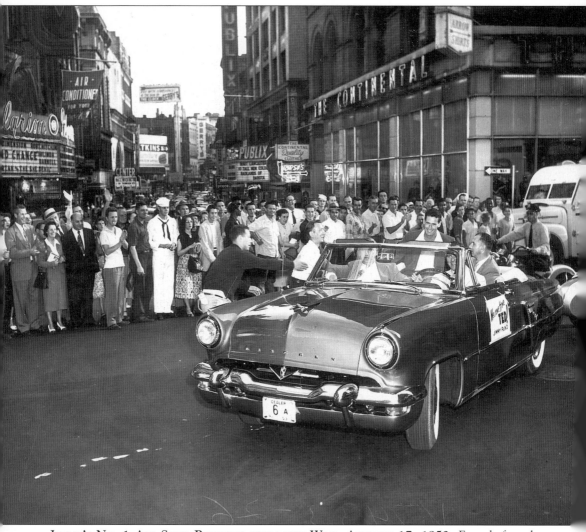

JIMMY'S NO. 1 ALL-STAR RETURNS FROM THE WAR, AUGUST 17, 1953. Even before the Jimmy Fund was the official charity of his team, Red Sox superstar Ted Williams had been one of its most prominent backers, making unsolicited appearances at theater collection drives and children's bedsides. By the time he returned in the summer of 1953 from a year serving as a Marine pilot in the Korean War, the Boston Braves had left town and the Red Sox had assumed their Jimmy Fund duties. When a welcome-home dinner in Williams' honor was planned at the Hotel Statler, Williams told Bill Koster, "If you make it $100-a-plate, with the proviso that everybody, and I mean *everybody*, has to pay, and all the proceeds go to the Jimmy Fund, I'll be there." Koster complied, and the Variety Club and Red Sox took care of the rest—starting with this motorcade through town. (Brearley Collection.)

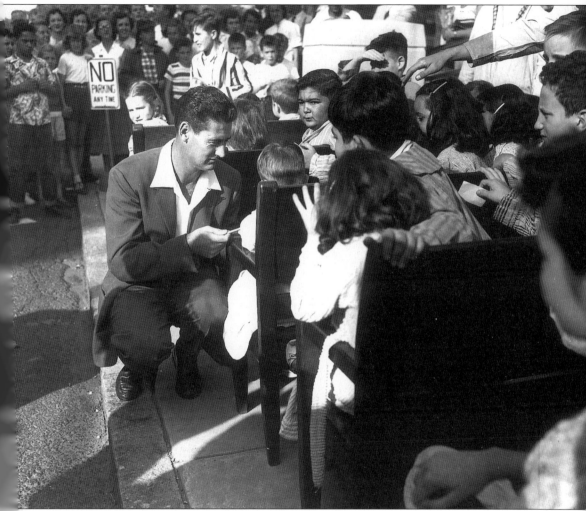

FIRST STOP—JIMMY FUND, AUGUST 17, 1953. Before heading to the hotel, the motorcade stopped at the Jimmy Fund Building on Binney Street. Young patients from the Jimmy Fund Clinic and Children's Hospital next door were seated on benches in the sunshine, where Williams took time to speak with them individually and sign autographs. Ed Sullivan, host of the popular television show *Toast of the Town,* joined Williams in meeting the kids and later accompanied him to the dinner, where he served as co-toastmaster with Red Sox broadcaster Curt Gowdy. Other evening attendees included Tom Yawkey, Lou Perini, Red Sox general manager Joe Cronin, and the entire Red Sox team. The program's theme was a simple one: "Three Strikes to Strike Out Cancer in Children." (Brearley Collection.)

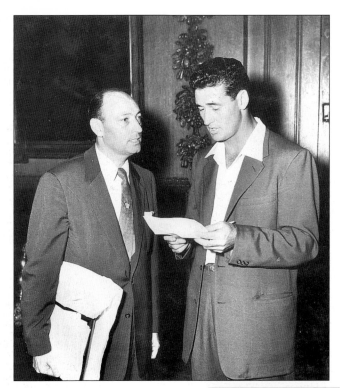

BILL KOSTER AND TED WILLIAMS REHEARSING THE BIG SPEECH, AUGUST 17, 1953. Despite his engaging personality, Williams was generally shy by nature and not a fan of making speeches. The words he prepared with Bill Koster (left) for the banquet were nonetheless powerful. "The way I look at it, there is always something we can do for some youngster somewhere," he said. "Here, we don't have to look any further than the Jimmy Fund." (Brearley Collection.)

A NIGHT FOR TIES, AUGUST 17, 1953. Williams (left) has had a lifetime abhorrence to neckties, and before this evening, reporters could remember only one occasion (in 1947) at which he had worn one. Out of deference for the Jimmy Fund and the coast-to-coast television audience, however, Williams donned a dark-blue tie before accepting the Variety Club's annual Great Heart Award for humanitarianism from Sidney Farber and Bill Koster (behind microphones). (Brearley Collection.)

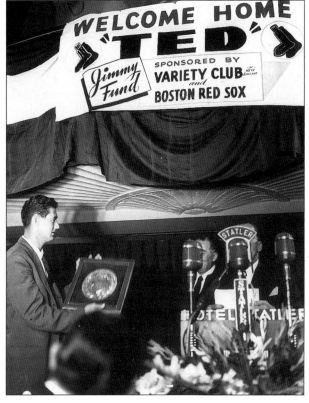

42

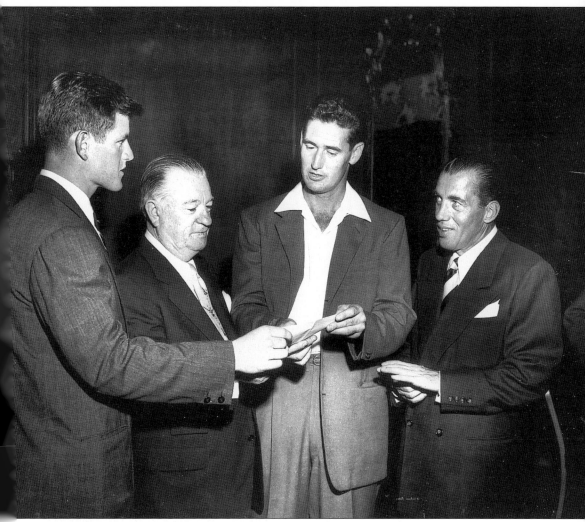

YOUNG EDWARD M. KENNEDY PRESENTS A SURPRISE GIFT, AUGUST 17, 1953. The climax to the evening came when 21-year-old Edward M. Kennedy handed Williams a $50,000 check from the Joseph P. Kennedy Jr. Foundation as Children's Cancer Research Foundation president Martin Mullin (second from left) and Ed Sullivan looked on. The unexpected gesture from the future Massachusetts senator brought the night's final tally to more than $125,000 collected for the Jimmy Fund in support of the Children's Cancer Research Foundation. It also marked the start of an ongoing bond between Boston's foremost political family and charity—a relationship that would include the cancer treatment of Edward M. Kennedy's own son in the early 1970s. Notice that Williams has already removed his dreaded tie. (Brearley Collection.)

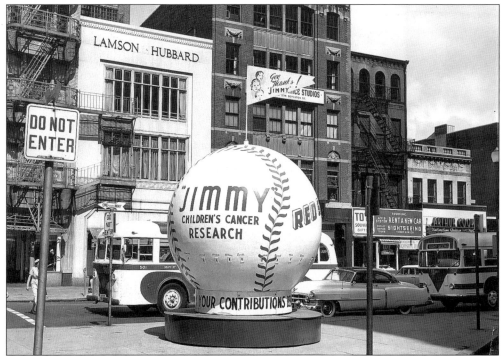

A JIMMY BALL OUTSIDE THE HOTEL STATLER, SEPTEMBER 1953. Among the most popular Jimmy Fund collection canisters were those made to resemble baseballs. This 10-foot-tall version was first used at Braves Field and was later placed outside the home office of the Variety Club in Boston's Hotel Statler. Fans encountering it were encouraged to vote for their favorite Red Sox player by placing coins in the slot by his name. (Jimmy Fund.)

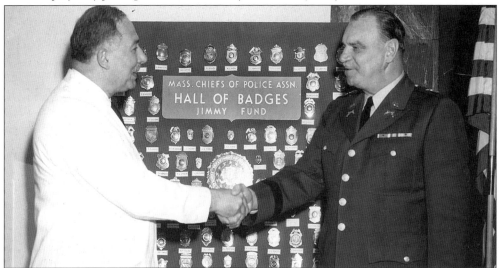

POLICE CHIEFS ANSWER THE CALL, 1956. Like the Red Sox, the Massachusetts Chiefs of Police Association made the Jimmy Fund its official charity in 1953. The Hall of Badges behind Sidney Farber (left) and Maj. Gen. William H. Maglin, provost general of the United States, is on display at Dana-Farber today. It holds shields from chiefs throughout the Commonwealth committed to the cause through fundraising efforts. (Boston Herald.)

SPENCER TRACY, JIMMY FUND THEATER PROGRAM PITCHMAN, THE 1950S. During the 1950s, top Hollywood stars such as Spencer Tracy, Joan Crawford, and James Cagney supported the Jimmy Fund/Variety Club Theatre Collections Program by producing movie trailers shown to audiences throughout New England each summer. As ushers passed around Jimmy Fund collection canisters, Tracy thanked viewers in his 1954 short "for your continued support of this wonderful work." (Jimmy Fund.)

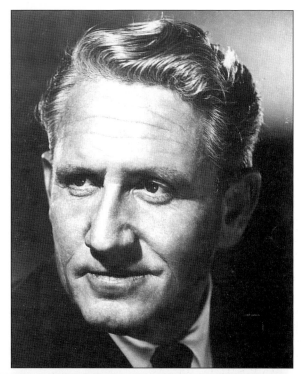

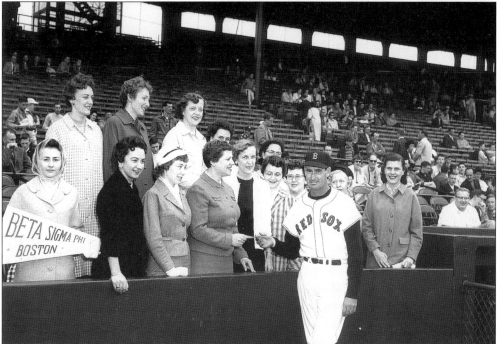

JUST ANOTHER DAY AT THE PARK, THE MID-1950S. Picking up checks for the Jimmy Fund became a regular pregame ritual at Fenway Park for Ted Williams and other Red Sox players during the 1950s, and the practice has continued to the present day. Here, Williams accepts a gift from the Beta Sigma Phi sorority, a longtime friend of the charity. (Jimmy Fund.)

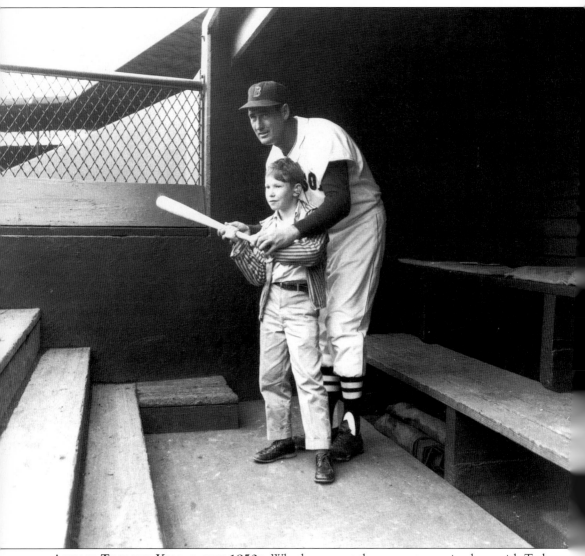

ALWAYS TIME FOR KIDS, C. THE 1950S. Whether or not the youngster posing here with Ted Williams at Fenway Park was a Jimmy Fund Clinic patient is unknown, but one thing is certain—he was the envy of all his friends. Scenes like this one were not often caught on film because Williams wanted no publicity surrounding his frequent meetings with kids—especially his visits to the Children's Cancer Research Foundation. Word spread of his generosity, however, and in time he became a one-man fundraising machine. Adults and children frequently approached him on the street with small donations, while others sent money to the Jimmy Fund for each home run he hit. "How nice it is to be on the same team with such wonderful people who have but one thought in mind—thinking of youngsters," Williams said in a 1950s interview. "Being part of the Jimmy Fund helps me as an individual in more ways than I can ever explain." (Brearley Collection.)

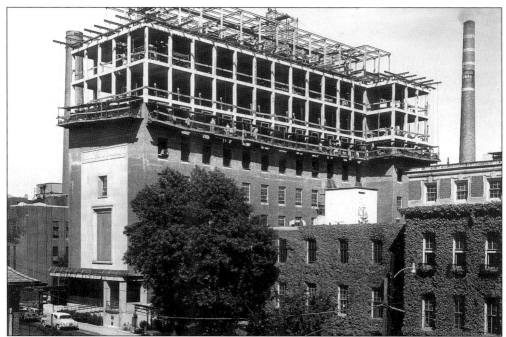

"THE HOUSE THAT JIMMY BUILT" GROWS TALLER, 1958. There is no more tangible sign of progress than the sight of girders reaching up to the sky, so when work began on four additional floors for the Jimmy Fund Building in the late 1950s, it was clear that Dr. Sidney Farber and his staff at the Children's Cancer Research Foundation were scaling new heights as well. Along with additional laboratory and storage facilities, the new space included a special suite for Farber on the top floor. (Jimmy Fund.)

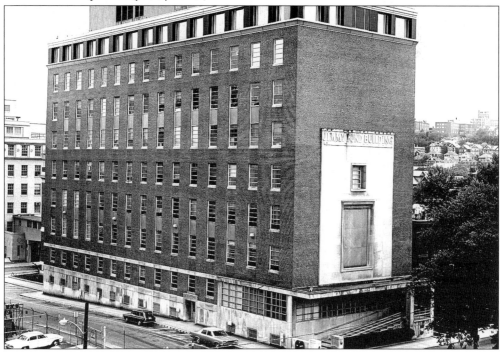

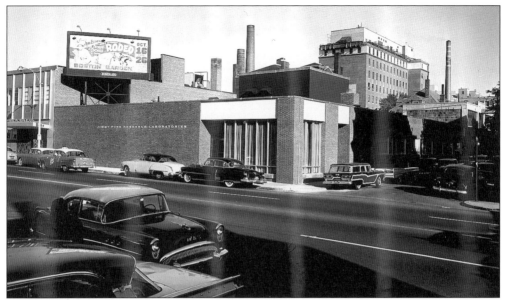

JIMMY FUND RESEARCH LABORATORIES OPEN, 1958. The newly enlarged Jimmy Fund Building looms in the distance of this photograph, which shows the Children's Cancer Research Foundation's second main facility around the time of its 1958 opening. Located at 462 Brookline Avenue, the Jimmy Fund Research Laboratories were designed primarily for the humane storage of thousands of mice and other research animals. The structure was eventually renamed the Arthur A. Redstone Animal Laboratories to honor a generous donor. (Jimmy Fund.)

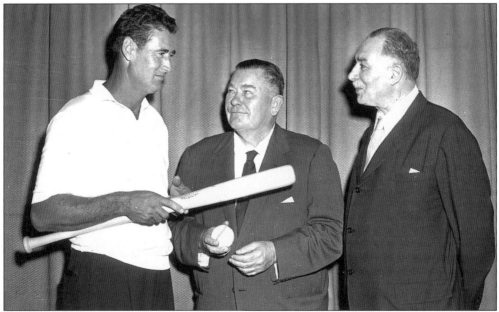

A TRIUMPHANT TRIO, AUGUST 1960. No three individuals played a bigger role in the explosive growth of the Jimmy Fund during the 1950s than Ted Williams, Tom Yawkey, and Dr. Sidney Farber. Williams was in the closing months of his fantastic Red Sox career when this photograph was taken, and it would end fittingly; after accepting a check for the Jimmy Fund before his last game, he homered in his final at-bat. (Brearley Collection.)

Three

A FORTUITOUS TRAIN RIDE AND CONTINUED GROWTH: 1962–1973

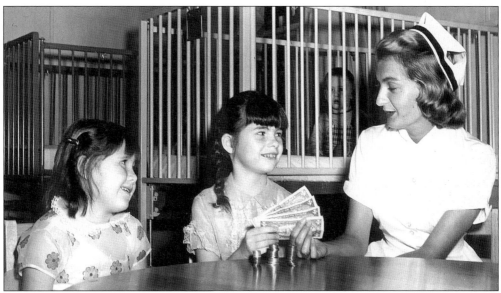

EVERY DOLLAR (AND NICKEL) COUNTS, THE EARLY 1960S. The Children's Cancer Research Foundation would receive many substantial gifts from individual and corporate donors during the 1960s, but grass-roots fundraising by the Jimmy Fund remained a crucial component of the foundation's growth. In this photograph, some youngsters do their part for the cause during a visit with Jimmy Fund Clinic nurse Barbara Powers. (Jimmy Fund.)

By the time it celebrated its 15th anniversary, the Children's Cancer Research Foundation (CCRF) had already made great strides in the battle against childhood cancer. Although aided by the tremendous fundraising efforts of the Jimmy Fund, Dr. Sidney Farber and his staff still needed additional financial support to continue their landmark research. In early 1961, Farber met a stranger while on a train, and by ride's end, that fellow passenger—Charles A. Dana Jr.—had become inspired by the scientist's enthusiastic quest.

Dana, in turn, told his father, industrialist Charles Dana Sr., about Farber's mission with the CCRF. Similarly impressed, the elder Dana and his wife, Eleanor, were moved to support the effort through the family's New York City–based philanthropic institution, which specialized in assisting health and educational causes. The first of many substantial gifts from the Charles A. Dana Foundation to the CCRF came the following year, and on November 30, 1962, the Charles A. and Eleanor N. Dana Laboratories were formally dedicated. The new $2.69 million laboratories in the Jimmy Fund Building cost twice the amount of the entire original five-story structure.

The Danas appreciated Farber's vision of blending biomedical research and patient care in a comprehensive facility and, in 1968, made another major gift of $5 million to help construct the Charles A. Dana Cancer Center on Binney Street, across from the Jimmy Fund Building. Through the years, the Dana Foundation has awarded a total of nearly $33 million in gifts to the foundation, which has since been renamed Dana-Farber Cancer Institute to recognize the family's generosity.

Today, the 17-story Dana building houses offices, laboratories, and clinics for both children and adults. An expansion of the CCRF's charter in 1969 enabled the foundation to treat patients of all ages, allowing everybody to benefit from Farber's philosophy of total patient care. David G. Nathan, M.D., who first worked with Farber at Children's Hospital in the early 1960s, remembers, "He decided that all services for the patient and family—clinical care, nutrition, social work, counseling—should be provided in one place. All decisions [about caregiving] should be made as a team."

Following this mission, the foundation grew in size and stature during the 1960s and early 1970s. As it did, the Jimmy Fund continued serving as the public face for the work being done by Farber and his staff. Fundraising efforts by celebrities—most notably the Boston Red Sox—continued. After Ted Williams was inducted into the National Baseball Hall of Fame in 1966, Jimmy Fund contributions poured in to honor the charity's "All-Time All-Star."

When the Red Sox startled the sports world by emerging from a decade near last place to capture the 1967 American League championship, they elevated New England's love affair with baseball to a new level that has never subsided. As record numbers of fans began to follow the team's exploits in person and on radio and television, the charity's name also resounded more than ever through pregame check ceremonies and the Jimmy Fund billboard atop the right-field grandstands of Fenway Park. For many years, this was the only advertising Tom Yawkey allowed in the park, and people came to expect its presence like an old friend.

CCRF executive director Bill Koster was another constant at Fenway, where he encouraged a new generation of players—from superstars like Carl Yastrzemski to rookies like Mike Andrews—to get involved by befriending young cancer patients. Koster arranged for all of the Jimmy Fund's on-field events, and he supplied Ken Coleman and the Red Sox broadcasting crew with a steady stream of salutes. They, in turn, followed in the tradition of announcers Jim Britt and Curt Gowdy by routinely pitching the charity over the airwaves during games.

Down the street from Fenway, Farber became a strong voice for strengthening the nation's commitment to cancer research. His status as a compelling speaker on the subject led to frequent appearances on Capitol Hill, where he forged bonds in Congress, met with Presidents Johnson and Nixon, and served on Johnson's Commission on Heart Disease, Cancer, and Stroke. Between 1957 and 1967, thanks largely to Farber's advocacy work, the annual budget for the National Cancer Institute—the government's primary funding arm for cancer study—increased from $48 million to $176 million.

In a letter dated the day before his assassination, Massachusetts native Pres. John F. Kennedy expressed his appreciation for Farber and the efforts of the CCRF. "This center, the first of its kind," he wrote, "has made a significant contribution to the nation's fight against cancer through the care, treatment, and study of cancer-stricken children. Your achievements have given new hope to many young patients and their families and have strengthened the promise that science will one day triumph over malignant diseases."

Even as his own health declined with heart attacks in 1965 and 1969 and a bout with cancer that few knew about, Farber continued seeing patients and leading his foundation's research agenda. In his mid-60s, he was named president of the American Cancer Society, and he maintained his belief that single treatments could be found for all cancers.

Eventually, Farber was forced to give up much of his demanding schedule. He retired from the Harvard Medical School faculty on September 1, 1970, and became professor emeritus after 41 years of service. To drum up financial support for the CCRF, he depended more than ever on Koster, the man known to many as "Mr. Jimmy Fund." In addition to helping garner contributions for the Dana building's construction, Koster nurtured the charity's many "fans," including its three mainstays: the entertainment industry, Major League Baseball, and the Massachusetts Chiefs of Police Association. "My father used to say the Jimmy Fund was like a three-legged stool," Koster's son Stephen P. Koster has recalled. "If we lose one leg, the stool falls."

The resolve of the elder Koster and his partner to conquer disease was embodied in the green-marble statuette of a raven on the side of Farber's otherwise clutter-free desk. The bird's head—pointed ever upward—symbolized hope to its owner, who once wrote, "Whenever a member of my staff, or the parents of a patient, feel despondent, I ask them to study it, and I think it helps them. There is much strength and beauty in it."

Farber did not see to its end his goal of a new cancer center on the CCRF campus. Shortly before the Dana building's completion, he died in his Jimmy Fund Building office on March 30, 1973, at the age of 69. He was mourned not only as one of the world's great physicians, but as a man who brought his lofty dream of a world without cancer far closer to reality than many had deemed imaginable a few decades before.

Advances at the Children's Cancer Research Foundation between 1962 and 1973 include the following:

> In 1963, CCRF investigators develop means to collect, preserve, and transfuse blood-clotting factors called platelets to control bleeding, a critical step to combating this common side effect of cancer chemotherapy.

> In 1969, the foundation's charter is expanded to provide services for patients of all ages.

> In work beginning in 1972 and continuing over three years, researchers are able to increase the cure rate for a bone cancer known as osteogenic sarcoma from less than 15 percent to more than 60 percent. Use of chemotherapy in addition to surgery or radiation therapy reduces many tumors to operable size and may even render surgery unnecessary.

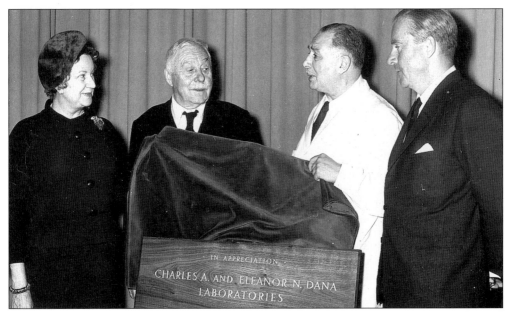

DEDICATION OF THE DANA LABORATORIES, NOVEMBER 30, 1962. An attorney who had served as a New York state legislator, Charles A. Dana later made his fortune in the automobile industry. Upon his retirement in 1950, he and his wife, Eleanor, founded the Charles A. Dana Foundation to create philanthropic programs that advance health and higher education. Impressed by Dr. Sidney Farber's wisdom and determination, the couple gave a substantial grant to the Children's Cancer Research Foundation (CCRF) for expansion of the laboratory facilities in the Jimmy Fund Building. Here, on dedication day, the Danas (left) mark the occasion with Dr. Farber and their son, Charles A. Dana Jr. (Jimmy Fund.)

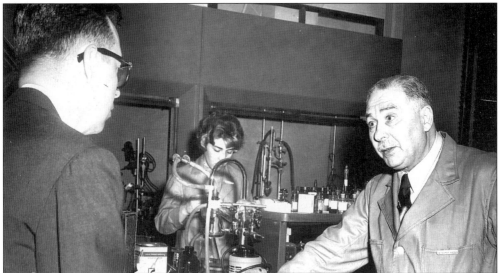

FARBER REFLECTS ON CANCER RESEARCH PROGRESS, MAY 1962. By the early 1960s, Farber and his staff were developing the means to collect, preserve, and transfuse blood-clotting factors called platelets to control bleeding, a common side effect of chemotherapy. Due to these and other advances, recovery rates for many forms of childhood cancer were increasing. In this interview with a Boston television reporter, Farber discusses the CCRF's progress. (Jimmy Fund.)

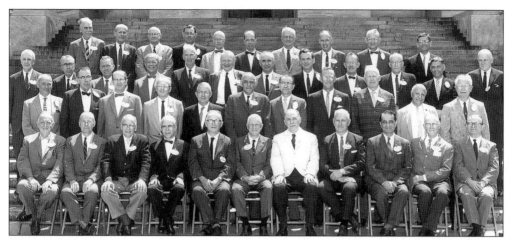

A Short Walk to the Reunion, June 1, 1962. When the Harvard Medical School Class of 1927 held its 35th reunion, Dr. Sidney Farber (first row, seventh from left) did not have far to travel. His office in the Jimmy Fund Building was a five-minute walk to his alma mater's campus. (Jimmy Fund.)

Dr. Sidney Farber and Cardinal Cushing, the Early 1960s. Archbishop of Boston Richard James Cushing was an early supporter of the Jimmy Fund and Farber. After Cushing's elevation to cardinal in 1958, he continued to be a strong advocate for the Children's Cancer Research Foundation. He was fond of referring to the Jimmy Fund as the "charity of the little man." (Boston Herald.)

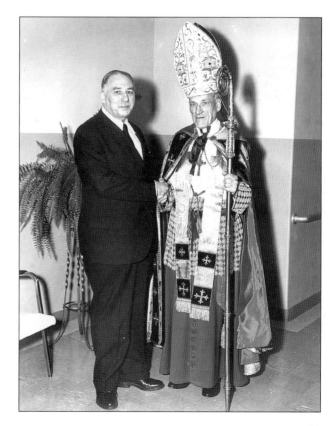

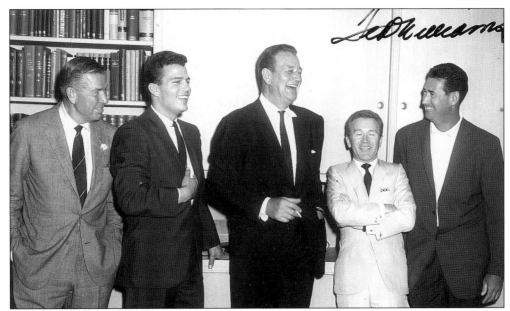

TWO LEGENDS MEET IN FARBER'S OFFICE, JUNE 26, 1962. In Boston after filming the African safari movie *Hitari!*, actors Bruce Cabot (far left), John Wayne (center, beside his son) and Red Buttons (fourth from left) stopped by the Jimmy Fund Building. There, in Dr. Sidney Farber's office, they happened upon another distinguished visitor—baseball great Ted Williams. It was the first time that Wayne and Williams had ever met. (Jimmy Fund.)

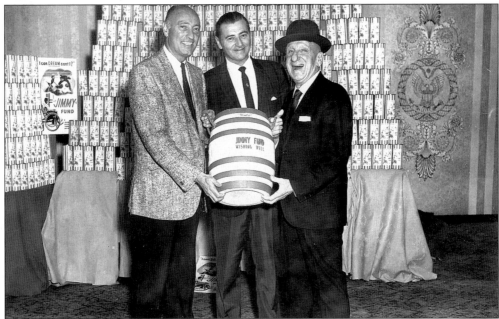

A NOSE FOR CHARITY, C. THE 1960S. The Jimmy Fund continued to depend on celebrity support to spread its message throughout the 1960s. Here, comedian Jimmy Durante (right) helps Bill Koster (left) and Koster's longtime assistant George Patenaude promote an effort by New England banks to have citizens turn in their change to benefit the Jimmy Fund and help alleviate a regional coin shortage. (Jimmy Fund.)

BRINGING HOPE TO THE JIMMY FUND CLINIC, C. THE 1960S. This time, Bob Hope is the guest getting a tour of the Jimmy Fund Clinic with Bill Koster (left) and Dr. Sidney Farber (right). The ongoing involvement of the Variety Club and the motion picture industry with the Jimmy Fund assured that such high-profile visits would go on. (Jimmy Fund.)

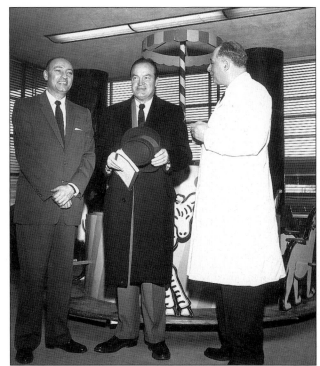

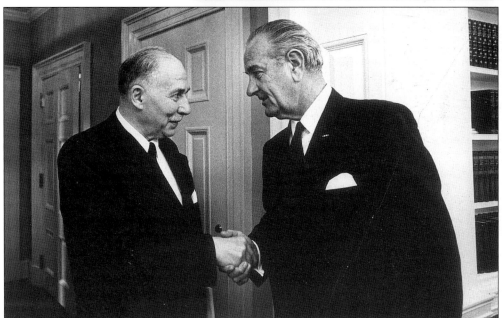

APPEALING TO LYNDON B. JOHNSON, 1965. Farber established strong political ties in Washington, D.C., during his career, making frequent speeches before Congress and the occasional White House visit in pursuit of increased national support for cancer research and treatment. In addition to lobbying Pres. Lyndon B. Johnson for a redoubled effort in these areas, he also served on Johnson's Commission on Heart Disease, Cancer, and Stroke in 1964–1965. (Jimmy Fund.)

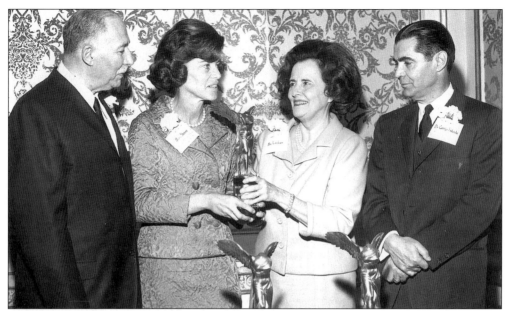

SHARING LASKER AWARD HONORS, 1966. Established after World War II, the prestigious Albert Lasker Medical Research Awards celebrate scientists, physicians, and public servants who have made advances in fighting diseases. These 1966 honorees are, from left to right, Dr. Sidney Farber, Eunice Kennedy Shriver (receiving a public service statuette for her work on behalf of mentally handicapped people), Mary Woodward Lasker, and molecular biologist Dr. George Palade. (Jimmy Fund.)

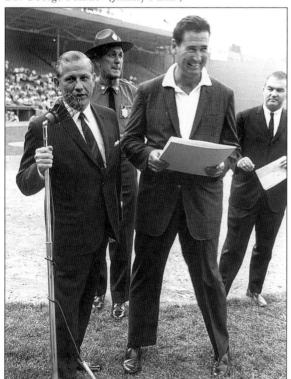

THANKING A HALL OF FAMER, JUNE 1966. When Ted Williams was inducted into the National Baseball Hall of Fame in 1966, fans honored the achievement by making record numbers of donations to the Jimmy Fund. In this photograph, Williams (center) is saluted before a Red Sox–Atlanta Braves Jimmy Fund exhibition game at Fenway Park by Massachusetts governor John A. Volpe while Sox broadcaster (and future Jimmy Fund director) Ken Coleman looks on. (Boston Herald.)

JEAN YAWKEY DOES THE HONORS, JUNE 1966. Red Sox owner Tom Yawkey's wife, Jean, presents Ted Williams with a plaque listing many of the friends and dignitaries who contributed to the special Jimmy Fund drive following Williams' Hall of Fame induction. A larger version of the plaque today resides in a gallery at Dana-Farber Cancer Institute that chronicles the institute's history and salutes Williams for his role in it. (Jimmy Fund.)

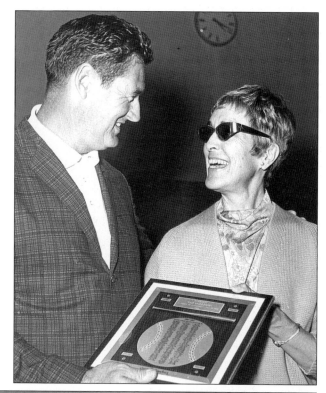

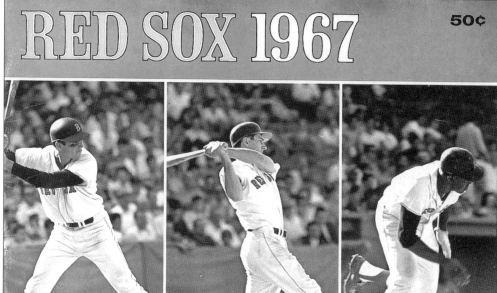

THE "IMPOSSIBLE DREAM" RED SOX GIVE JIMMY HIS SHARE, 1967. After finishing in ninth place the previous year, the 1967 Boston Red Sox captured an improbable American League championship. When it came time to divide up the club's World Series bonus money, captain Carl Yastrzemski suggested the players honor owner Tom Yawkey and give a full share of $5,000-plus to the Jimmy Fund. Although many of his teammates made less than $20,000 in annual salary, they agreed unanimously. (New England Sports Museum.)

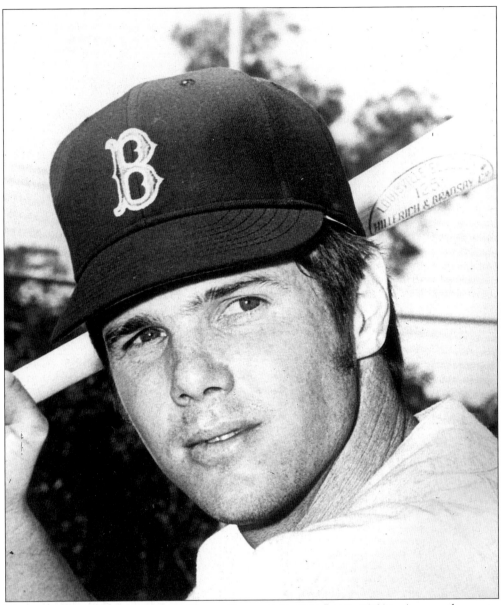

MIKE ANDREWS, FUTURE JIMMY FUND CHAIRMAN, THE LATE 1960s. Among the many players to help the 1967 Red Sox to the World Series was 23-year-old rookie second baseman Mike Andrews. One day that season, a chance meeting with a young Jimmy Fund patient set his post-playing career in motion. "Bill Koster was always out at the ballpark, getting players to meet with kids undergoing cancer treatment," Andrews recalls. "One day a teammate got stuck in the trainer's room, so Bill asked me to take his place. I was busy warming up, but I talked for a few minutes to the kid, who was a Little League star looking forward to playing the next year. I wished him luck. Bill came up to me afterwards and said, 'Thanks, Mike, that meant a lot. There isn't much we can do for that boy. We're sending him home.' That made me realize that a hitless day at the plate didn't mean much in the scheme of things." This exchange paved the way for Andrews' decades-long involvement with the Jimmy Fund, the last 23 years as its chairman. (Jimmy Fund.)

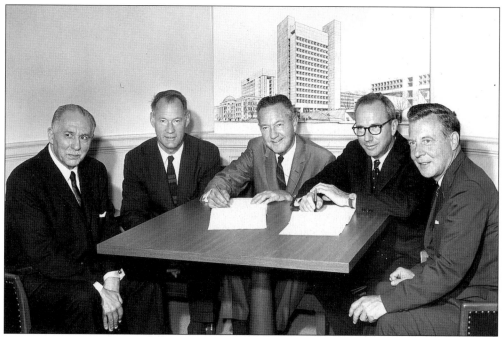

THE CHILDREN'S HOSPITAL ALSO GROWS, SEPTEMBER 1967. While the Children's Cancer Research Foundation continued to prosper and prepare for physical expansion in the late 1960s, Dr. Sidney Farber was also heavily involved with securing a new Basic Pediatric Sciences Building for Children's Hospital. Here, Farber (far left) and fellow representatives from both the hospital and the construction firm slated to build the 17-floor structure sign a contract for the project. (Boston Herald.)

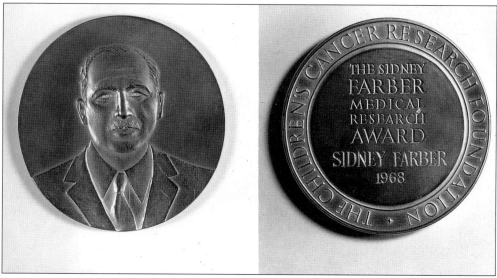

A FITTING TRIBUTE, 1968. After numerous other honors, Farber received the distinction of having one named for him in 1968. The Sidney Farber Medical Research Award, established by the Children's Cancer Research Foundation, is given to those individuals or groups "who have made significant contributions to medical science, or to its development, furtherance, and support." Appropriately, Farber himself was the first recipient. (Jimmy Fund.)

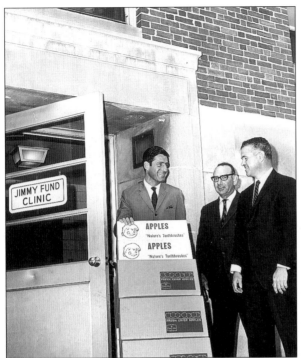

ANOTHER DELIVERY FOR MORT LEDERMAN, APRIL 1968. Mort Lederman (left) joined the Children's Cancer Research Foundation as an administrative assistant in 1952. In a half-century of unparalleled service, he has held various key positions, including manager of General Services and security director. Lederman enjoyed an especially close relationship with Sidney Farber, to whom he often leant paperback mystery novels. In this view, Lederman accepts an edible donation from members of the Massachusetts Department of Agriculture. (Jimmy Fund.)

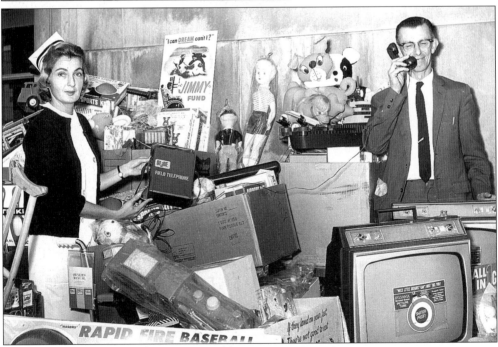

PRESENTS APLENTY, THE LATE 1960S. Apples are not the only non-monetary items given to the Jimmy Fund over the years. Toys, stuffed animals, board games, televisions, and much more have made their way into the thankful hands of youngsters and adults challenged by a cancer diagnosis. Here, Jimmy Fund Clinic nurse Barbara Powers helps a visitor call for reinforcements on a G.I. Joe phone after a barrage of gifts lands at the clinic door. (Jimmy Fund.)

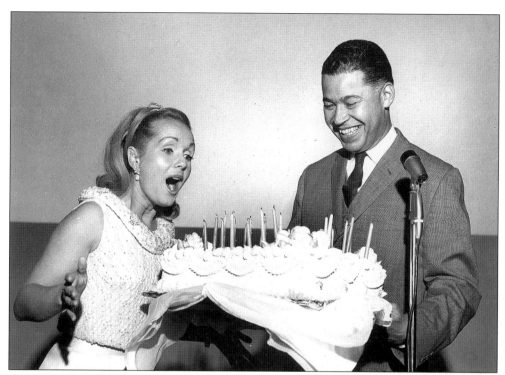

TURNING 21 IN STYLE, 1968. Helping to blow out the candles at a 21st birthday party held for the Children's Cancer Research Foundation are actress Debbie Reynolds and Massachusetts senator Edward Brooke. Reynolds is among the long list of film stars who have made appeals for the Jimmy Fund over the years. (Jimmy Fund.)

TED KENNEDY SALUTES SIDNEY FARBER, 1969. After Dr. Sidney Farber was named president-elect of the American Cancer Society, he was honored with a dinner at Anthony's Pier 4 restaurant in Boston. The featured speaker (dining with him here) was one of Farber's most devoted advocates: Sen. Edward M. Kennedy. Two decades later, Kennedy would receive the Sidney Farber Medical Research Award for his career-long allegiance to health-care issues, including federally funded cancer research. (Jimmy Fund.)

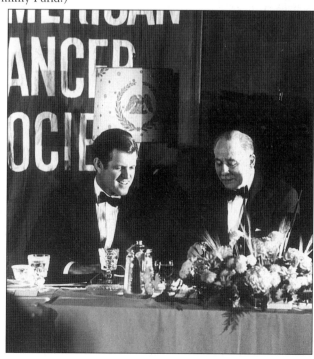

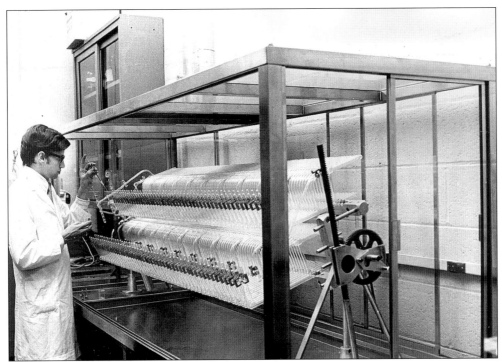

RESEARCH CONTINUES, 1969. State-of-the-art equipment like this system used for the purification of peptides enabled scientists at the Children's Cancer Research Foundation (CCRF) to continue seeking cancer breakthroughs. By 1969, when the foundation expanded its charter to provide services for patients of all ages, plans were already well under way for construction of a new 17-floor research facility on the CCRF campus. (Jimmy Fund.)

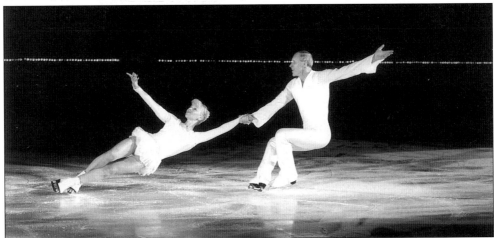

"AN EVENING WITH CHAMPIONS" FULFILLS A SKATER'S DREAM. During a visit to Children's Hospital in Boston for a routine knee examination in 1970, Harvard College student and figure skater John Misha Petkevich had a chance encounter with some young cancer patients. Moved by the experience, he started his own annual event to support the Jimmy Fund. Combining the efforts of student volunteers from Harvard's Eliot House and the world's most celebrated skaters (including Olympians Oleg and Ludmila Protopopov, shown here), "An Evening with Champions" is still going strong after 30-plus years. (Steve Gilbert photograph.)

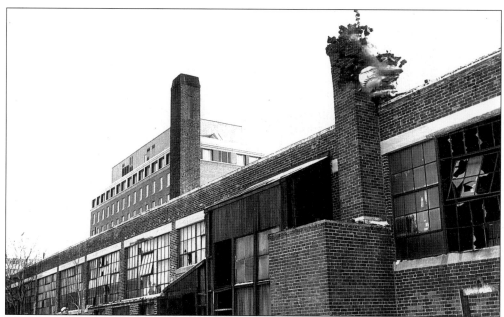

MAKING WAY FOR THE DANA CANCER CENTER, 1970. Constructing the CCRF's new $10 million facility a few feet from the Jimmy Fund Building required first razing the existing structure on the site—the old Boston Schoolbook Depository. A wrecking ball decorated to resemble a baseball was an appropriate tool for the job, as money collected for the Jimmy Fund by the Boston Red Sox over the years had helped make such a project possible. (Jimmy Fund.)

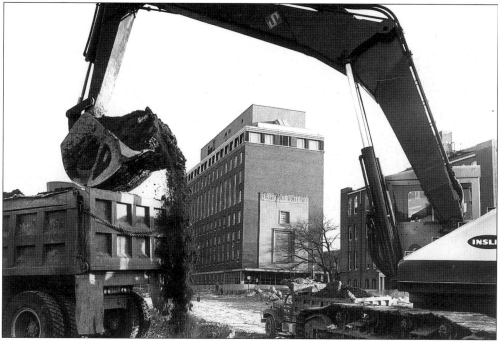

LOOKING (AND DIGGING) TO THE FUTURE, C. 1970. The Jimmy Fund Building is a silent spectator as bulldozers get to work creating room for the 17-floor Charles A. Dana Cancer Center. (Jimmy Fund.)

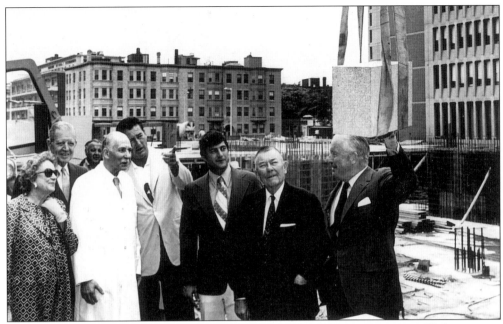

CORNERSTONE CEREMONIES DRAW AN ALL-STAR CROWD, JUNE 29, 1971. Within a year, work on the Dana Cancer Center had progressed enough to hold a cornerstone ceremony. Representing the Dana family, whose foundation had already granted $5 million toward the project, with more to come, are Eleanor (far left) and Charles A. Dana Jr. (far right). Joining them are, from left to right, Dr. Sidney Farber, Ted Williams, Carl Yastrzemski, and Tom Yawkey. (Jimmy Fund.)

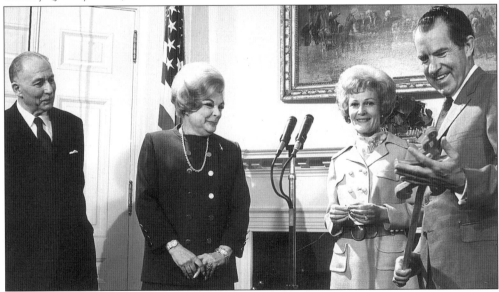

FARBER HELPS THE NIXONS MARK WAR ON CANCER, 1971. Dr. Sidney Farber (far left) was a White House guest of Pat Nixon (third from left) and Pres. Richard Nixon (far right) after the president declared his "war on cancer" and passed the National Cancer Act of 1971. When the president appointed 18 members to a National Cancer Advisory Board the following March, Farber was granted a four-year term. (Jimmy Fund.)

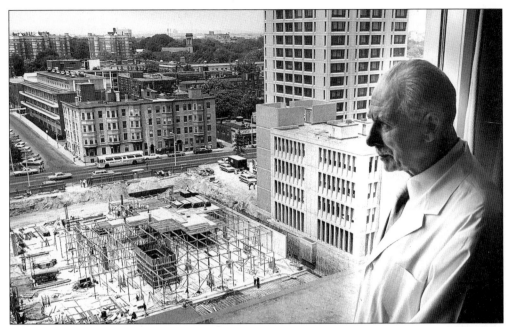

WATCHING HIS DREAM CONTINUE TO GROW, 1972. Looking out from his office windows on the top floor of the Jimmy Fund Building, Dr. Sidney Farber could watch construction progress on the Charles A. Dana Cancer Center across the street. The building represented the embodiment of Farber's dream for a comprehensive cancer facility. (Boston Herald.)

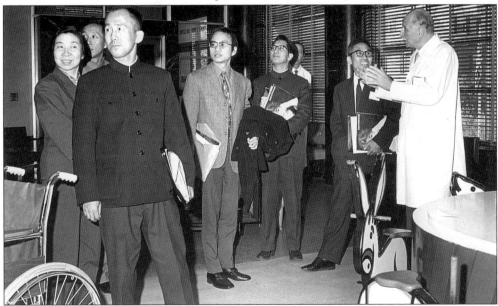

A TIRELESS WORKER, SEPTEMBER 1972. Even as his 69th birthday came and went, an exuberant Farber could often be seen leading dignitaries around the Children's Cancer Research Foundation campus when not conducting his own research. In this view, he takes a Chinese delegation on a tour of the Jimmy Fund Clinic; a few months later, he played host to Dr. Natasha Perevodchikova—one of the Soviet Union's leading cancer chemotherapists. (Jimmy Fund.)

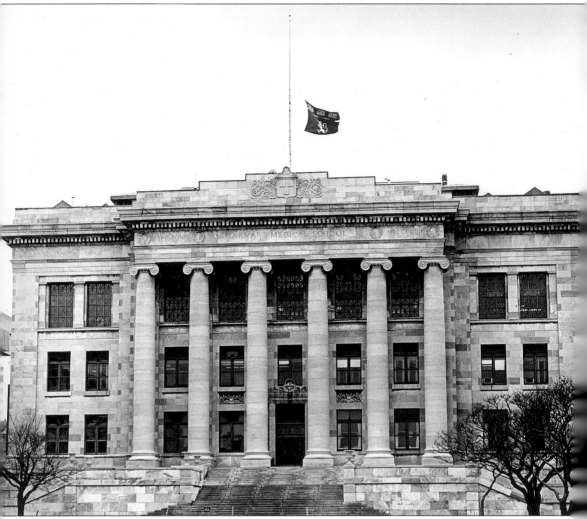

HARVARD AND THE MEDICAL WORLD MOURN FARBER'S DEATH, APRIL 1973. On March 30, 1973, Dr. Sidney Farber died at his Jimmy Fund Building desk. While he had been in declining health, his death at age 69 still sent shockwaves through the medical world. Newspaper stories mourned his passing as a major blow to cancer research and recounted his incredible career accomplishments and nine honorary degrees. As his wife, Norma, and his four children held a private funeral, the flag flew at half-mast over Harvard Medical School (above) one block from the Children's Cancer Research Foundation campus he had built to prominence. "Dr. Farber's Life Over, But His Work Continues" read a headline in Boston's *Sunday Herald Advertiser*.

"The spirit of this great medical statesman deserves to live on, and it will live on. It will live on in every hospital and research institution where men and women work to stamp out the disease of cancer."

—Bill Koster, Jimmy Fund Auditorium memorial service, May 13, 1973

Four
DR. FARBER'S LEGACY: 1973–1989

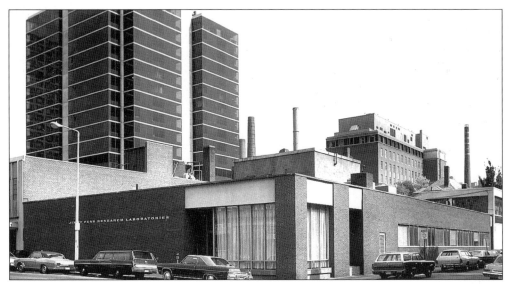

THE CHARLES A. DANA CANCER CENTER RISES ABOVE THE SFCC CAMPUS, C. 1976. In this photograph taken from across Brookline Avenue, the newly completed Charles A. Dana Cancer Center rises majestically above the other buildings on the campus of Sidney Farber Cancer Center (SFCC). The 17-floor facility was formally dedicated on June 28, 1976, at a ceremony featuring speeches from Sen. Edward M. Kennedy and Stephen B. Farber, son of SFCC founder Sidney Farber. (Jimmy Fund.)

Just as the entire nation underwent a period of dramatic change during the early 1970s—with war continuing in Vietnam and the Watergate scandal unfolding in Washington—the Children's Cancer Research Foundation (CCRF) was also in a state of transition. Its founder and leader of 25 years, Dr. Sidney Farber, had died in March 1973. His goal of establishing the CCRF as one of the world's foremost cancer centers had become a reality, but now that center needed someone new at its helm.

Enter Dr. Emil Frei III. Recruited to the foundation as physician-in-chief the previous year from M.D. Anderson Cancer Center in Houston, Frei was known for co-developing the world's first treatment leading to a complete cure for leukemia patients. With his colleague Emil Freireich, M.D., he had also pioneered the revolutionary approach of combination chemotherapy—considered one of the most important advances in cancer treatment in the last quarter of the 20th century. Like Farber, Frei was actively involved in pushing for passage of the National Cancer Act of 1971.

Just nine months after his arrival in Boston, Frei assumed leadership of the CCRF upon Farber's death. As director, he continued his predecessor's mission by recruiting some of the world's finest physician-scientists and overseeing completion of the Charles A. Dana Building. With this new research and treatment facility, the foundation expected to boost annual outpatient visits from 20,000 to more than 50,000. It could also offer inpatient adult care for the first time, thanks to 64 new acute-care beds.

During Frei's first year at the helm, the CCRF changed its name to the Sidney Farber Cancer Center (later Institute) to honor its late founder. It also brought another Farber onto its full-time staff: Darwin Farber, Dr. Farber's youngest brother. After a career spent building hospital clinics, Darwin Farber was named director of planning and development at the CCRF, where he oversaw completion of the Dana building and a staff increase from 200 to 1,000 in just two years. He still serves the institute today as a trustee.

The Jimmy Fund also experienced major transition during this period. In the mid-to-late 1970s, it lost two of its most important figures with the passing of CCRF executive director Bill Koster and Red Sox owner Tom Yawkey. Koster had led the Jimmy Fund from its 1948 inception and had raised approximately $53 million for the cancer center. Yawkey, winner of the Sidney Farber Medical Research Award in 1973 for outstanding contributions to the fight against cancer, had helped expand the Jimmy Fund's popularity by maintaining it as his team's official charity for more than two decades. Ironically, both Yawkey and Koster died of cancer.

Both these individuals, however, would have worthy successors. Upon Tom Yawkey's death, Red Sox ownership went to a group including his wife, Jean; in the years that followed, she would keep the Jimmy Fund tradition alive at Fenway Park. The team's connection to the cause extended onto the charity's own staff as well, with longtime Sox broadcaster Ken Coleman taking over Koster's role as Jimmy Fund executive director.

Coleman and his staff spearheaded the development of widely popular and profitable events during this period. The Jimmy Fund Golf Program, which today boasts more than 150 annual tournaments, officially debuted in 1983, the same year as the Scooper Bowl—the world's largest annual ice-cream festival. Ski events, radiothons, and a cross-state "Run for Jimmy" by the Massachusetts Chiefs of Police Association also became regular calendar events. When Coleman stepped down in the mid-1980s, former Red Sox infielder Mike Andrews—another longtime Jimmy Fund volunteer—took his spot leading the charity, a role he still holds today.

The Jimmy Fund Council of Greater Boston, a group comprised of volunteers, was founded in 1977 and, over the next two decades, hosted a series of "Jimmy Fund Tributes" for such sports stars (and friends of the charity) as Red Auerbach, Bobby Orr, Carl Yastrzemski, and Marvin Hagler. The largest and most successful was "An Evening with Ted Williams No. 9 and Friends," a sold-out, $200-a-plate dinner at Boston's Wang Center for the Performing Arts in honor of Williams' 70th birthday in 1988. Another critical all-volunteer group, the Friends of Sidney Farber Cancer Institute, began supporting research and patient care in 1976. Today, it boasts 1,700 members.

The most successful annual event to start during this era was the Pan-Massachusetts Challenge (PMC), a two-day, 192-mile bike-a-thon first wheeled out in 1980. Started by Billy Starr in memory of his mother, who died of cancer, it grew from 36 participants and $10,200 collected in its first year into the Jimmy Fund's single largest fundraising event today. In 2001, the PMC drew more than 3,100 cyclists (including 160 cancer survivors) and presented a check for $14 million to Dana-Farber.

Nineteen eighty was a watershed year off-road as well. Frei shed his presidential duties to concentrate on clinical issues as physician-in-chief, and Baruj Benacerraf, M.D., succeeded him as president. Benacerraf, then also chairman of the Department of Pathology at Harvard Medical School, received the Nobel Prize for Physiology or Medicine that December for his pioneering studies of the human immune system. During the course of his presidency (through 1992), Benacerraf would create a results-oriented work environment that placed equal importance on patient care, research, and teaching. Physical improvements during his tenure included a complete overhaul of the Jimmy Fund Research Laboratories in 1981 and construction of the state-of-the-art Louis B. Mayer Research Laboratories, which opened in 1988.

In the midst of all this transition, the Sidney Farber Cancer Institute was renamed Dana-Farber Cancer Institute in 1981 to recognize the generous support of the Charles A. Dana Foundation—which marked the occasion with a $10 million gift. Such benevolence helped the center to achieve extraordinary results by decade's end: two of every three children who entered the Jimmy Fund Clinic, and more than half of all people with cancer, were being cured.

Research achievements at DFCI during the 1970s included the following:

Designation in 1973 as a regional Comprehensive Cancer Center by the National Cancer Institute.

Discovery of the first-known cancer-causing gene, or oncogene.

Pioneering the use of multiple drugs (combination chemotherapy) in the treatment of cancer.

Increased cure rates for some forms of adult non-Hodgkin's lymphoma, osteogenic sarcoma (a form of bone cancer), and soft-tissue sarcomas.

Improved survival rates for patients with acute lymphocytic leukemia (ALL), breast cancer, and advanced testicular cancer.

Breakthroughs in the 1980s included the following:

Designation as New England's only Center for AIDS Research by the National Institute of Allergies and Infectious Diseases.

Development of autologous (self) bone-marrow transplantation as a treatment for childhood leukemia.

Discovery that the immune system is turned "on" by helper T cells and "off" by suppressor T cells. The AIDS virus infects and destroys helper T cells, eventually rendering its host defenseless against disease.

Development of a new generation of anti-cancer drugs, called immunotoxins, which deliver a potent poison to cancer cells and leave normal cells unscathed.

Identification of the growth-controlling role of the gene RB-1 and other "tumor-suppressor" genes.

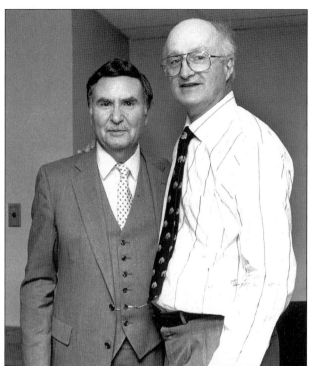

DARWIN FARBER AND DR. EMIL FREI III. Named director of the Children's Cancer Research Foundation upon Dr. Sidney Farber's death in 1973, Dr. Emil Frei III (right) was able to maintain his predecessor's high standards of research and clinical excellence while expanding the foundation's physical plant in the years that followed. Among those aiding him in these efforts was director of planning and development Darwin Farber, Dr. Farber's brother. In 1997, this duo would co-chair Dana-Farber's 50th anniversary festivities. (Jimmy Fund.)

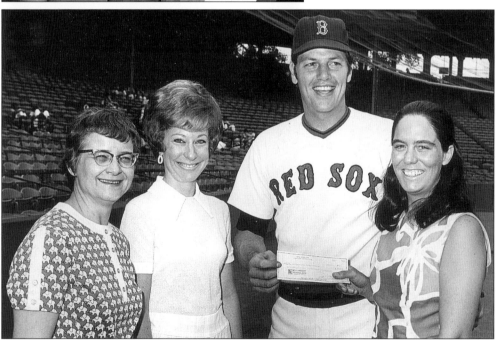

CONTINUING THE FENWAY TRADITION, C. THE 1970S. In a scene similar to that on page 45, Boston Red Sox catcher and New Hampshire native Carlton Fisk accepts a Jimmy Fund gift at Fenway Park from a new generation of Beta Sigma Phi sorority sisters. As the charity neared its 30th anniversary, Red Sox players like Fisk were still there to pick up a check or visit patients in the Jimmy Fund Clinic. (Jimmy Fund.)

THE FAMILIAR FENWAY LANDSCAPE, THE
LATE 1970S. Fenway Park in Boston is best
known for the Green Monster—its 37-foot-
high left-field wall. Most New Englanders,
however, are also well acquainted with
another spot in the old ballpark: the right-
field grandstands. It is there, on the roof,
that a billboard advertising the team's
official charity—the Jimmy Fund—has
stood for as long as many people can
remember. (Jimmy Fund.)

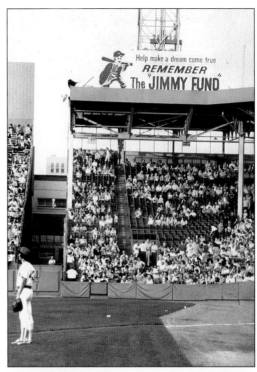

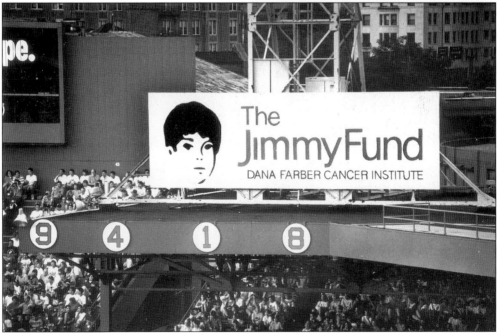

JIMMY GETS A FACELIFT, C. 1989. The images have changed a bit over the years, but the
message remains the same: this is Jimmy's team. For many years, the Jimmy Fund billboard was
the only advertisement Red Sox owner Tom Yawkey allowed in his ballpark, and when the Red
Sox decided to post their retired uniform numbers, they were placed by Fenway's most hallowed
spot. (Steve Gilbert photograph.)

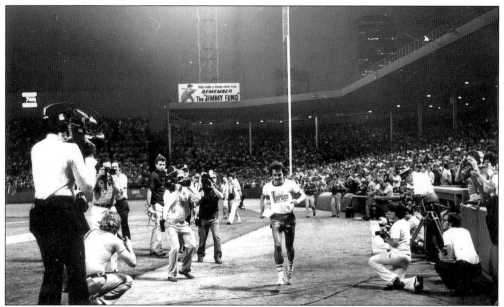

DAVID MCGILLIVRAY, THE 3,400-MILE MAN, 1978. Of all the individual fundraising feats undertaken to raise awareness for the Jimmy Fund, perhaps none was more grueling than what David McGillivray pulled off in 1978. Starting in Medford, Oregon, on June 11, he ran 3,400 miles across the country over 80 days—finishing at Fenway Park on Jimmy Fund Night (August 29). The next day, 1,500 people mailed $19,607.63 to the charity in his honor. (Jimmy Fund.)

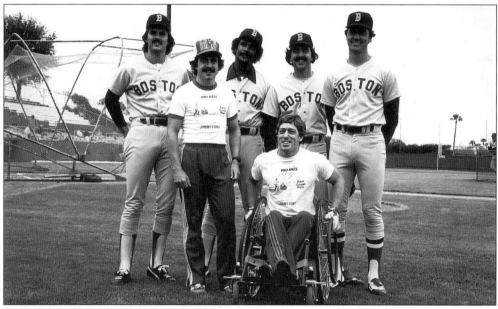

A WINTER HAVEN SEND-OFF, FEBRUARY 1980. Less than two years later, McGillivray (second from left) was at it again—this time with Boston Marathon wheelchair champion Bob Hall. After a send-off from these Red Sox players at their Florida spring-training complex, the pair trekked 1,520 miles up the East Coast over 38 days to reach Boston's Copley Square. The players are, from left to right, Dennis Eckersley, Jim Rice, Dick Drago, and Dwight Evans. (Jimmy Fund.)

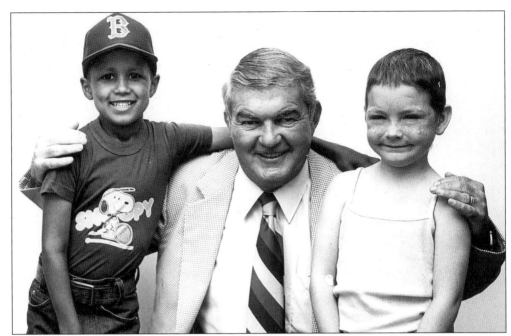

KEN COLEMAN COMES ABOARD, 1978. For the first 29 years of the Jimmy Fund's existence, Bill Koster was its only director. When he decided to step down in 1977, the charity did not have to look far for a successor. Red Sox broadcaster and Quincy, Massachusetts native Ken Coleman (shown here with some young friends) had been a loyal Jimmy Fund volunteer for more than a decade, and he stepped smoothly into the leadership role. (Jimmy Fund.)

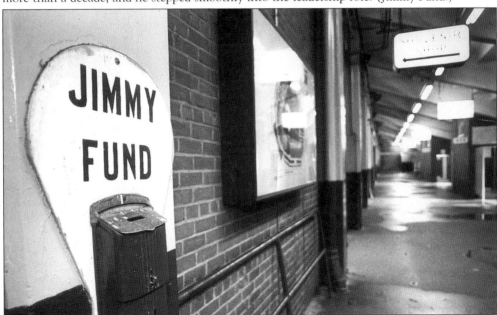

JIMMY FUND COLLECTION BOXES AT FENWAY PARK, THE LATE 1970S. Another familiar sight at Fenway Park are the mailbox-style Jimmy Fund collection boxes affixed to posts throughout the interior of the ballpark. Although a bit antiquated in design, the boxes have done their duty well for decades. (Jimmy Fund.)

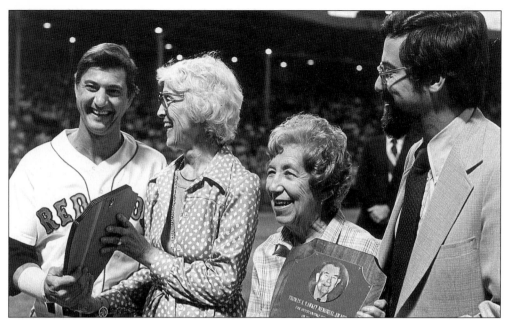

CARL YASTRZEMSKI AND BILL KOSTER NAMED FIRST YAWKEY AWARD WINNERS, SEPTEMBER 1979. As a tribute to the late Boston Red Sox owner, the Jimmy Fund established the annual Thomas A. Yawkey Memorial Award in 1979 for outstanding service of 10 years or more to the charity. Considered the Jimmy Fund's highest honor, it went first to Red Sox great Carl "Yaz" Yastrzemski (left, getting his award from Jean Yawkey) and (posthumously) to longtime Jimmy Fund director Bill Koster. Rae Koster accepted her late husband's plaque with help from son Stephen. (Jimmy Fund.)

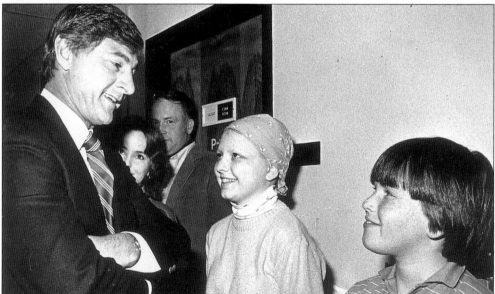

SHARING A SMILE WITH CAPTAIN CARL, 1984. Like Ted Williams, whom he succeeded in left field for the Red Sox, Carl Yastrzemski has a natural way with children and a soft spot for the Jimmy Fund. Here, shortly after his retirement, he shares a moment with Jacquelyn Manzi and Patrick Gormely outside the Jimmy Fund Clinic. (Jimmy Fund.)

GIVING JIMMY THE SHIRT(S) OFF HIS BACK, OCTOBER 1983. Few people at Fenway Park for Carl Yastrzemski's final game with the Boston Red Sox in 1983 will ever forget the emotional moment when Yaz spontaneously circled the ballpark and shook hands. Most of the spectators did not know, however, that Yastrzemski changed his uniform jersey after each inning that day and then donated all 10 shirts to the Jimmy Fund to auction off. (New England Sports Museum.)

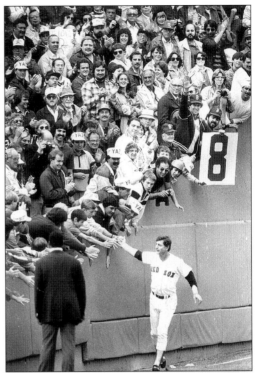

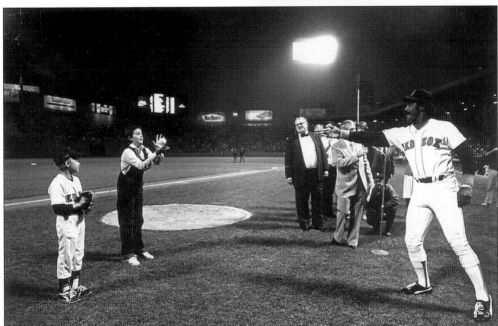

JIM RICE CONTINUES THE MOST VALUABLE PLAYER TRADITION, THE EARLY 1980s. In being named honorary chairman of the Jimmy Fund in 1979, Jim Rice was carrying on the legacy established by fellow Red Sox superstar left fielders Ted Williams and Carl Yastrzemski. Here, Rice tosses a ball to 14-year-old Susan Fennel of the Jimmy Fund Clinic for first-pitch duties at Fenway Park while 8-year-old Kevin Stefanek patiently waits his turn. (Jimmy Fund.)

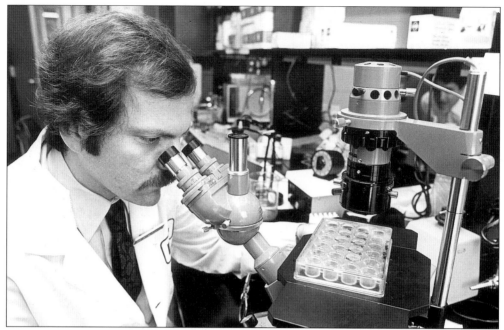

RESEARCH EFFORTS REACHING NEW HEIGHTS, 1981. Bolstered by the recruitment and development of an impressive corps of young physician-scientists during the 1970s and early 1980s—including Dr. Steven Burakoff, shown here—Dana-Farber continued to build upon its reputation as a stellar research institution. When new challenges such as AIDS arose, DFCI investigators were among those at the forefront of meeting them. (Jimmy Fund.)

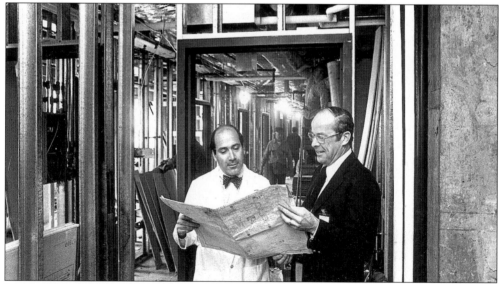

JIMMY FUND RESEARCH LABS UNDERGOING RENOVATIONS, 1979. As the Jimmy Fund Building neared its 30th anniversary, work began on completely renovating its research laboratories. Here, Dr. David Livingston (left), chairman of the institute's Biohazard Control Committee, and Thomas MacNamara, director of Support Services and Construction, inspect the progress under way on the seventh floor. The "rededication" of the building came on May 31, 1981, after three years and $6.3 million in costs. (Jimmy Fund.)

DR. BARUJ BENACERRAF RECEIVES THE NOBEL PRIZE, 1980. Dana-Farber's new president, Dr. Baruj Benacerraf (left), bolstered the institute's worldwide recognition in 1980 when he was awarded the Nobel Prize for Physiology or Medicine for the discovery that genetic factors play a role in determining the strength of an individual's immune system. After receiving his award from King Carl XVI of Sweden, Benacerraf donated his entire $72,000 portion of the prize money to Dana-Farber. (Jimmy Fund.)

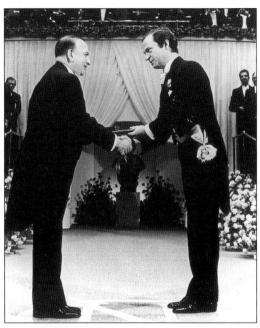

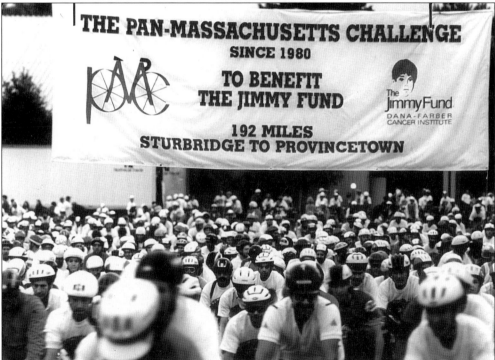

PAN-MASSACHUSETTS CHALLENGE RIDERS PEDAL FOR PROFITS, 1988. On a summer day in 1980, Billy Starr jumped onto the back of a pickup truck in Springfield, Massachusetts, and shouted to 35 friends, "Let's go! See you in Plymouth." Thus began the first Pan-Massachusetts Challenge (PMC) bike-a-thon, founded by Starr to honor the memory of his mother. The inaugural 140-mile ride raised $10,200 for the Jimmy Fund; through Starr's drive and leadership, the 1988 PMC (above) collected nearly $900,000. (Jimmy Fund.)

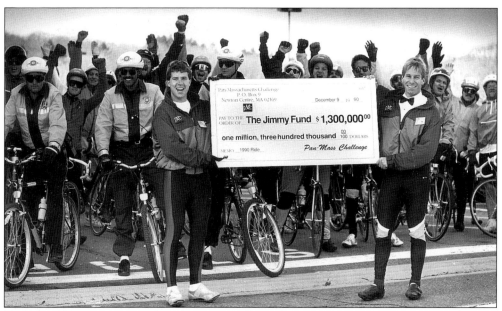

THE PAN-MASSACHUSETTS CHALLENGE AND BILLY STARR SURGE AHEAD, 1990. By the time it reached its 10th anniversary, the Pan-Massachusetts Challenge (PMC) bike-a-thon was garnering more than $1 million annually for the Jimmy Fund. When the 1990 ride took in a record $1.3 million, event founder Billy Starr (right, holding check) and assistant Chris McKeown (left) took a chilly celebration ride through Newton with about 100 fellow PMCers. (Boston Herald.)

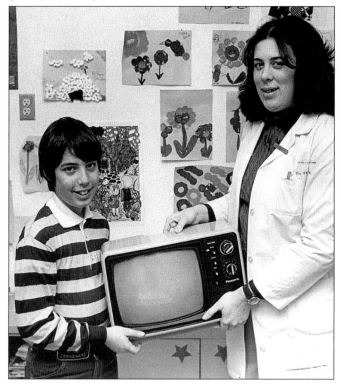

A LITTLE PEDDLER DOES HIS PART, 1978. Riding in the PMC is not the only way cyclists can help the Jimmy Fund. When 11-year-old Saul Kaplan of Lexington (left) won a television set for collecting the most money ($206.19) of anybody under 16 in the 1978 American Cancer Society bike-a-thon, he donated his reward—a new television set—to head nurse Peggy McCabe, R.N., of the Jimmy Fund Clinic for kids there to enjoy. (Jimmy Fund.)

BLUE EYES AND THE GREEN MONSTER, C. 1981. After Frank Sinatra performed a sold-out Boston concert that raised $110,000 for the Jimmy Fund in 1981, he was given a unique souvenir by two Jimmy Fund Clinic patients: a piece of Fenway Park's fabled Green Monster. The Red Sox had resurfaced their famous 37-foot-high left-field fence after the 1975 season, and pieces of the old wall were sold to fans for contributions to the Jimmy Fund. (Jimmy Fund.)

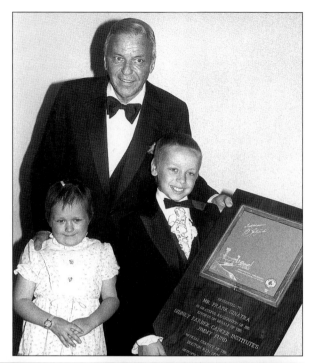

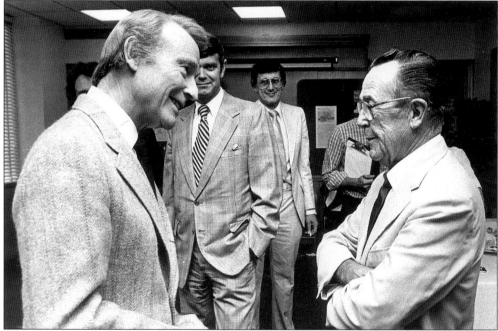

RALPH EDWARDS MAKES HIS FIRST CLINIC VISIT, SEPTEMBER 4, 1981. More than 30 years after his radio interview with a 12-year-old cancer patient launched the Jimmy Fund, *Truth or Consequences* host Ralph Edwards (left) finally saw the results of what he had helped start. After touring the Dana-Farber campus and meeting with staff members, including Dr. George Foley (right), Edwards was honored at Fenway Park that night as a recipient of the Yawkey Award. (Jimmy Fund.)

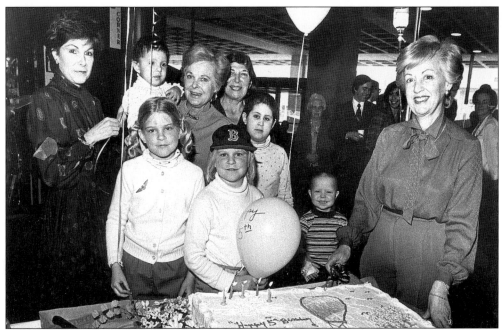

"FRIENDS CORNER" CELEBRATES FIVE YEARS OF SERVICE, 1983. Starting with a $200 grant and a handful of dedicated women in 1976, the Friends of Dana-Farber Cancer Institute has grown into a 1,700-member all-volunteer organization that has raised more than $13 million for vital research and patient care. The Friends Corner Gift Shop, opened in the Dana building in 1978, remains a favorite shopping spot for patients and their families. (Jimmy Fund.)

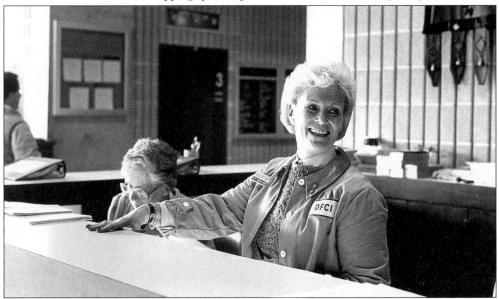

FIFI SWERLING KELLEM, A FRONT DESK FIXTURE, C. THE 1980S. During the 1970s, Fifi Swerling Kellem's daughter Susan was treated at Dana-Farber for ovarian cancer. When Susan died at age 20 in 1975, her mother felt she wanted to give something back to the institute and began volunteering at the front desk of the Dana building. For more than 20 years since, her smile has been the first thing many patients see when arriving for treatment. (Jimmy Fund.)

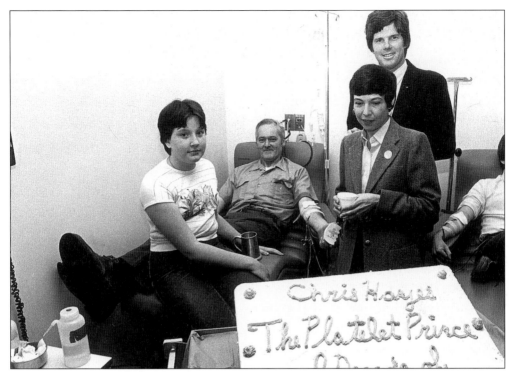

CHRIS HAYES, "PLATELET PRINCE," JUNE 1982. Another person compelled to thank the institute for care his child received is Chris Hayes, Dana-Farber's all-time platelet donor champion. When Hayes (in chair) reached his 10th anniversary of donating the life-saving blood-clotting agents in 1982, his wife, Clare, daughter Maura, and Mike Andrews of the Jimmy Fund helped him celebrate. By 2002, Hayes had made more than 750 platelet donations. (Jimmy Fund.)

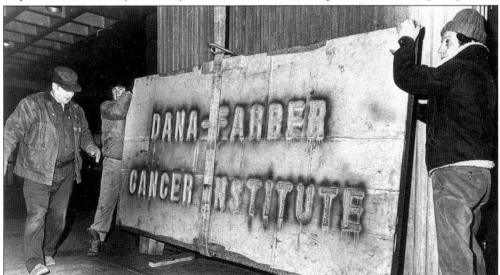

A NEW NAME HONORS TWO LEADERS, 1983. In recognition of significant contributions made by industrialist-philanthropist Charles A. Dana and his family foundation, Sidney Farber Cancer Institute was renamed Dana-Farber Cancer Institute in 1983. The Charles A. Dana Foundation marked the occasion with a $10 million grant to Dana-Farber. (Jimmy Fund.)

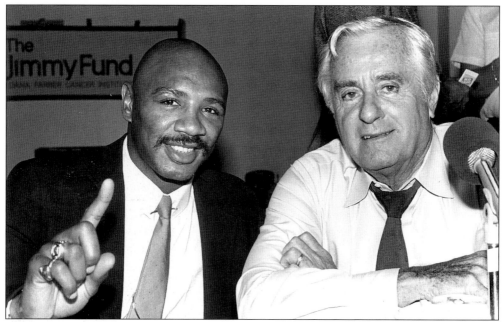

"MARVELOUS" MARVIN HAGLER AND CURT GOWDY AT THE JIMMY FUND RADIOTHON, AUGUST 1985. Chairman Mike Andrews and a variety of celebrity hosts—including World middleweight boxing champion "Marvelous" Marvin Hagler (left) and legendary Red Sox broadcaster Curt Gowdy—went on the air starting in 1984 during annual one-day Jimmy Fund Radiothons. The popular fundraisers, which were transmitted throughout New England over the Campbell Sports Network, collected more than $1.1 million in their first five years. (Steve Gilbert photograph.)

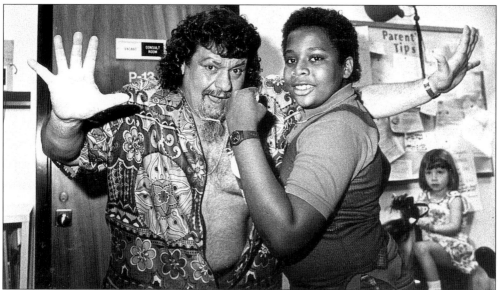

"CAPTAIN LOU" MAKES A JIMMY FUND CLINIC VISIT, JULY 1986. Another championship fighter who aided the cause during the 1980s was professional-wrestling king "Captain Lou" Albano, who took his licks from 12-year-old Jerrod Edwards during a 1986 visit to the Jimmy Fund Clinic. (Boston Herald.)

PRINCE CHARLES HAS A JOLLY GOOD VISIT, SEPTEMBER 3, 1986. Displaying his trademark charm and regular-guy manner, the Prince of Wales made a memorable trip to Dana-Farber in 1986. At the institute to show his interest in a program linking the United Kingdom with Dana-Farber Cancer Institute and Children's Hospital, the prince took time to speak with nearly every young patient he encountered—including 10-year-old Danny Casey (in dark coat). (Brad Herzog photograph.)

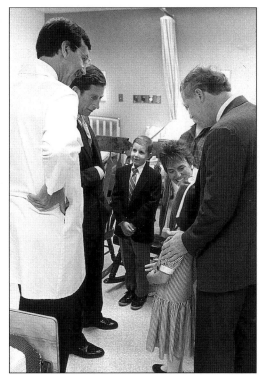

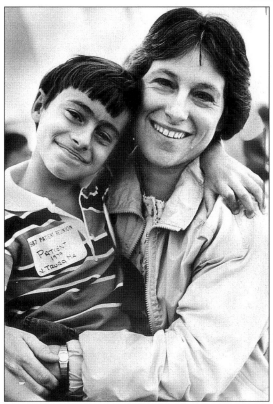

THE DANA-FARBER PATIENT REUNION, AUGUST 29, 1987. One of the most popular events during the 40th anniversary observances at Dana-Farber in 1987 was the institute's first-ever patient reunion. Approximately 175 pediatric and adult patients first treated at Dana-Farber at least five years before celebrated with their families and former caregivers, among them 10-year-old Eric Days and his mother, Cindy. (Boston Herald.)

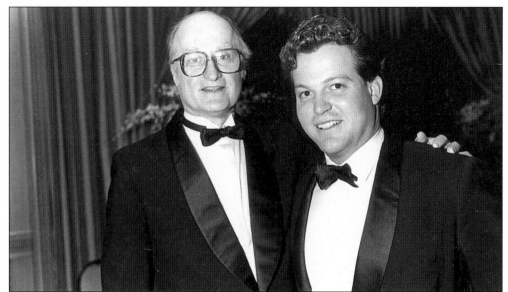

Dr. Emil Frei III and Former Patient Ted Kennedy Jr., 1988. In the fall of 1973, Sen. Edward M. Kennedy's son, 12-year-old Ted Kennedy Jr., was under the care of Emil Frei for a malignant bone tumor in his right leg. Young Ted survived after an amputation, and when Dana-Farber held a dinner honoring Frei's accomplishments 15 years later, Ted Jr. and Sr. were among the co-chairs. (Jimmy Fund.)

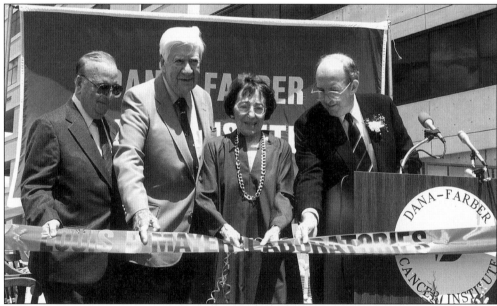

The Louis B. Mayer Laboratories Open, June 3, 1988. After movie giant Louis B. Mayer was treated for leukemia by Dr. Sidney Farber in 1957, he called him "the single most important man I have ever met." A $5 million grant from the Louis B. Mayer Foundation helped establish a new research facility at Dana-Farber. Shown at the 1988 dedication are, from left to right, DFCI president Baruj Benacerraf, M.D., House Speaker Thomas P. "Tip" O'Neill, Mayer's daughter Irene Mayer Selznick, and DFCI chairman of the board Vincent O'Reilly. (Steve Gilbert photograph.)

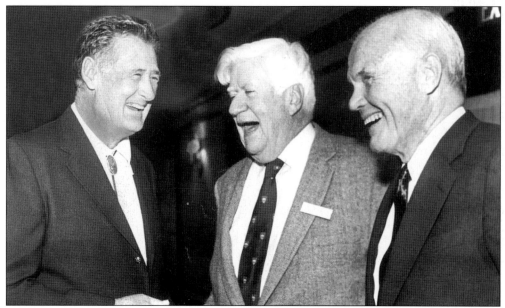

TWO PILOTS AND A POLITICIAN, NOVEMBER 10, 1988. In recognition of Red Sox legend Ted Williams' 70th birthday, the Jimmy Fund held a night in his honor at Boston's Wang Center for the Performing Arts in November 1988. "An Evening with Ted Williams No. 9 and Friends" raised $225,000 for the Jimmy Fund and gave the charity's No. 1 All-Star (left) a chance to catch up with old friends like House Speaker Tip O'Neill and Sen. John Glenn, with whom he flew jets in the Korean War. (Boston Herald.)

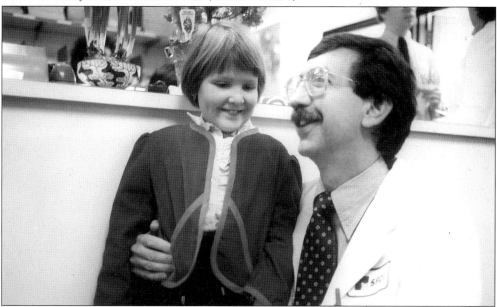

DR. SALLAN'S TOUCH, THE 1980S. Dr. Stephen E. Sallan joined the staff of Sidney Farber Cancer Institute in 1975 and has remained ever since. Today, he serves as Dana-Farber's chief of staff and is recognized as one of the world's foremost experts on childhood leukemia. His work has helped dramatically increase survival rates for the disease, and Jimmy Fund Clinic patients are big fans of his friendly smile and warm touch. (Jimmy Fund.)

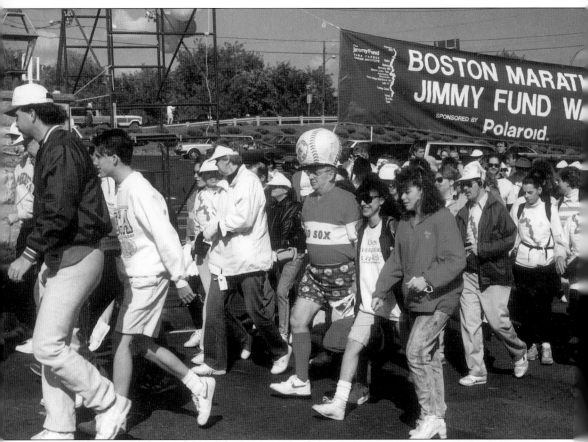

THE BOSTON MARATHON JIMMY FUND WALK DEBUTS, SEPTEMBER 23, 1989. Envisioning a fundraising event that families could take part in together, the Jimmy Fund held its first Boston Marathon Jimmy Fund Walk in 1989. Participants were able to traverse all or part of the famous 26.2-mile race course, and the day proved a huge success. The event has now raised more than $22 million since its inception, and in 2001 alone, nearly 8,500 people hoofed it for Jimmy. Over the years, inspirational signs and creative attire have become commonplace along the Hopkinton–Copley Square route. For instance, the man "having a ball" in the center of this photograph trekked the whole course for several years while wearing his distinctive Red Sox hat. (Jimmy Fund.)

Five

WHEELS, WALKS, AND
MORE OF PROGRESS:
1990–2002

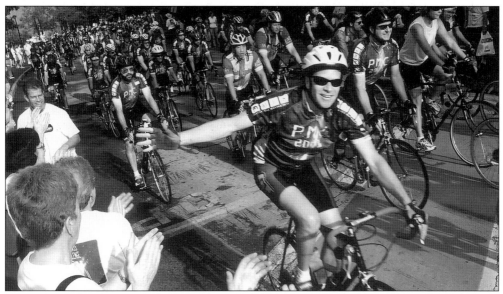

RIDING HIGH IN WELLESLEY, 2001. Record-breaking fundraising events have been a commonplace occurrence for the Jimmy Fund in recent years, with none more successful than the Pan-Massachusetts Challenge (PMC) bike-a-thon. This enthusiastic rider making crowd contact at the Wellesley start of the 2001 PMC was one of a record 3,100 participants that helped the two-day ride reach new heights. (Jimmy Fund.)

As the Jimmy Fund reached its 50th anniversary, this charitable arm of Dana-Farber Cancer Institute (DFCI) refined its fundraising formula by adding new events and building upon already successful ones. It set records annually for donor contributions and, in 1998, experienced one of the most dramatic moments in its history with the unexpected return of its namesake, Einar "Jimmy" Gustafson—a 62-year-old truck driver and former patient of Dr. Sidney Farber. Most had assumed Jimmy had died long ago from his childhood cancer.

Under the leadership of Mike Andrews, the Jimmy Fund saw an explosion in participation and contribution levels as New Englanders pounded pavement for the cause. While nearly 1,000 cyclists raised $1.4 million in the 1990 Pan-Massachusetts Challenge (PMC), the numbers had sped all the way to 3,100 riders and $14 million presented in 2001.

Fast on the heels of the PMC was the Boston Marathon Jimmy Fund Walk. It, too, experienced stellar growth, increasing its proceeds from $1 million in 1993 to $4 million in 2001. Despite coming just after the September 11 terrorist attacks, the 2001 walk drew nearly 8,500 participants, many of whom showed their patriotism with flags and red, white, and blue attire. Similar enthusiasm was exhibited for the Jimmy Fund Golf Program, which swelled from 20 tournaments in its inaugural season of 1983 to 150 tourneys held throughout the country in 2001. Each summer brought the Jimmy Fund/Variety Club Theatre Collections Program, firmly entrenched as the charity's longest-running event and still going strong in more than 200 cinemas and nearly 20 states.

As in past decades, new initiatives also emerged during this period. In 1991, the Jimmy Fund first partnered with Stop & Shop on its Triple Winner Program, in which Stop & Shop customers who make $1 contributions to the Jimmy Fund receive a scratch card with three chances to win up to $10,000 in cash. Co-sponsored by the Boston Red Sox, the program has become the Jimmy Fund's most successful corporate fundraiser and has helped pave the way for similar programs with Hyundai, Dunkin' Donuts, Burger King, and others.

Baseball and the Red Sox have maintained their strong connection to the Jimmy Fund. John Hancock Fantasy Day at Fenway, introduced in 1993, offers fans a chance to take batting practice in the team's famed home in exchange for support of the charity. The Ted Williams 406 Club, formed in 1995 to honor the Hall of Famer's stellar 1941 batting average, raised $2 million to fund a Ted Williams Senior Investigator at Dana-Farber. Since filling its initial 406 memberships, the club has been integrated into DFCI's annual leadership giving program.

When the Splendid Splinter returned to the institute in 1999, the electricity on campus reached an all-time high. In February 2002, as control of the Red Sox was shifting away from the Yawkey family for the first time since 1933, the new owners announced the club would continue its nearly 50-year relationship with the Jimmy Fund. "The Red Sox are a part of the fabric of this city, and the Jimmy Fund is an inseparable part of the Red Sox," said incoming team president and CEO Larry Lucchino, a cancer survivor who was treated at Dana-Farber in the mid-1980s.

Meanwhile, as the genetic revolution took shape between 1990 and 2002, the institute grew to keep at the forefront of new technology and maintain its leadership position in research. DFCI expanded its faculty and technology base to better understand the molecular workings of cells, and it opened two new research facilities—the Thomas A. Yawkey Laboratories in 1990 and the Richard A. and Susan F. Smith Research Laboratories in 1997. The latter facility had room for more than 500 Dana-Farber researchers, state-of-the-art laboratories, and an expanded library.

In addition to a time of physical expansion, it was also a decade of partnerships for the institute. In 1996, it formed Dana-Farber/Partners Cancer Care, a collaborative program in adult cancer care with Brigham and Women's Hospital and Massachusetts General Hospital. As part of this process, Dana-Farber's inpatient beds shifted over to Brigham and Women's, a move that allowed DFCI to focus on its outpatient services and develop specialized programs to meet the needs of patients with different kinds of cancers.

To strengthen cancer research efforts in the Harvard medical community, the institute spearheaded the 1999 creation of the Dana-Farber/Harvard Cancer Center, which encourages sharing among seven Harvard institutions. Also, DFCI formalized its more than 50-year relationship with Children's Hospital in 2000 with the creation of Dana-Farber/Children's Hospital Cancer Care. In this relationship, outpatient pediatric oncology care is delivered in the Jimmy Fund Clinic, and inpatient cancer care is provided at Children's Hospital.

Much of this evolution was led by DFCI's fifth president, David G. Nathan, M.D., a Boston native who remembers his uncle, Lou Gordon, meeting with other Variety Club members to help form the Jimmy Fund. Nathan attended Harvard Medical School as the Jimmy Fund and Children's Cancer Research Foundation were being developed and had later created one of the world's premier training programs in pediatric hematology and oncology.

After succeeding Prof. Christopher Walsh at Dana-Farber's helm in October 1995, Nathan guided the institute to a new level of prominence in patient safety, research, and treatment. He also oversaw the 50th anniversary celebrations of Dana-Farber and the Jimmy Fund.

In October 2000, Nathan was succeeded by one of his former students, Edward J. Benz Jr., M.D. An internationally recognized hematologist, Benz had chaired the Department of Medicine at Johns Hopkins University School of Medicine for five years. In succeeding his longtime mentor, he set goals for the decade ahead of making an impact on major common forms of cancer (lung, breast, colon, and ovarian cancers) through technology and teamwork, both locally and nationally.

"I think we need to help the public understand this is a fight we can win, but it's going to be a long and tough one," Benz said upon taking office. "Cancer is a bigger problem than Dana-Farber, Harvard, Partners HealthCare System, or even the National Cancer Institute. I think we'll measure our accomplishments by how we can be the lens that focuses resources on cancer and gets people working together."

Important clinical developments at Dana-Farber between 1990 and 2002 include the following:

Opening of the David B. Perini Jr. Quality of Life Clinic in 1992 to provide care to survivors of childhood cancers and conduct research to better understand the long-term effects of childhood cancer treatment.

Opening of the Gillette Center for Women's Cancers in 1997 to provide team-based care to patients with breast, ovarian, cervical, and other women's cancers.

Creation in 1999 of the Leonard P. Zakim Center for Integrated Therapies, which offers services such as acupuncture, massage, and meditation while conducting formal research into such therapies' effectiveness.

Development of the pioneering Patient and Family Advisory Councils, which recognize the important role patients and families can play in their care.

Research advances include the following:

Discovery of a flaw in a gene known as p53 that researchers use to demonstrate that susceptibility to developing cancer can be passed from one generation to the next.

Development with Columbia University investigators of the first three-dimensional picture of a protein that enables the human immunodeficiency virus (HIV) to infect cells of the immune system.

Discovery that a drug (Gleevec), which achieved striking success against chronic myelogenous leukemia, can shrink and even eliminate tumors in some patients with a rare and otherwise incurable form of gastrointestinal cancer called GIST.

The first human study of Endostatin (Protein), one of the angiogenic drugs now being tested for their effectiveness in cutting off the blood supply to tumors.

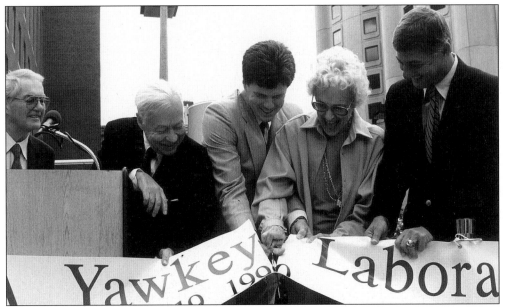

DEDICATION DAY FOR YAWKEY LABORATORIES, MAY 19, 1990. The 1990s got off to a great start at Dana-Farber as the institute dedicated the new Thomas A. Yawkey Laboratories in the Jimmy Fund Building. Helping Boston Red Sox owner Jean Yawkey, fourth from left, honor her late husband are, from left to right, Ken Coleman, former American League Baseball president Lee MacPhail, Mike Andrews, and Carl Yastrzemski. (Steve Gilbert photograph.)

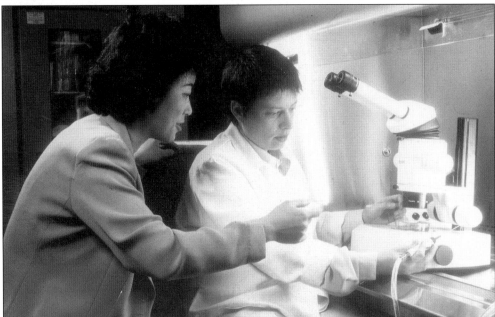

TECHNOLOGY FUELS NEW RESEARCH, THE 1990S. Both in the Yawkey Laboratories and at other research venues throughout the Dana-Farber campus, physician-scientists like Lynda Chin, M.D., (left) and Kornelia Polyak, M.D, Ph.D., have worked in recent years to take the exciting advances in genetic analysis made possible by emerging technology and make inroads toward cancer cures. (Sam Ogden photograph.)

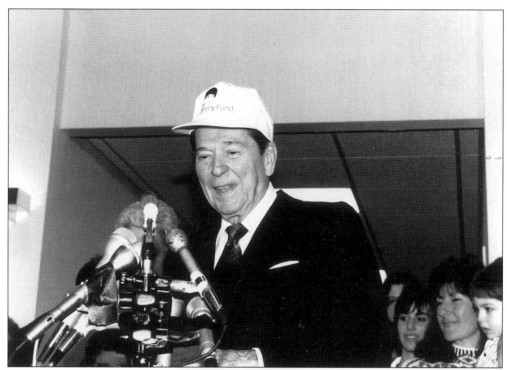

"The Gipper" and "The Greatest" Come to Dana-Farber Cancer Institute, the Early 1990s. Celebrity sightings at Dana-Farber on behalf of the Jimmy Fund continued into the new decade, including visits by a pair of the world's most recognizable and beloved figures: former president Ronald Reagan (1990) and former heavyweight boxing champion Muhammad Ali (1992). Both icons met with patients in the Jimmy Fund Clinic during their respective tours, and Reagan was also the guest of honor at a Sheraton Boston luncheon—with all proceeds going to the Jimmy Fund. (Steve Gilbert, Jimmy Fund photographs.)

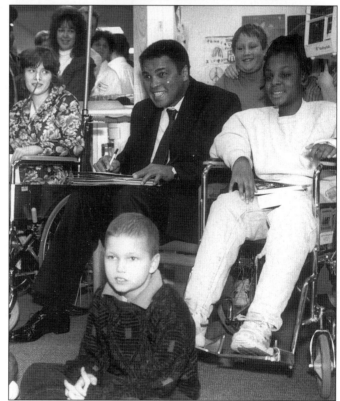

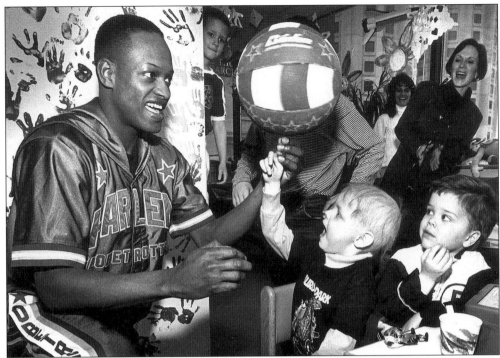

HAVING A BALL IN THE JIMMY FUND CLINIC, MARCH 1995. One never knows who is going to walk—or dribble—into the Jimmy Fund Clinic. Here, Robert Wallace of the Harlem Globetrotters puts the spin on Michael Fox's finger as Jeffery Crimins wonders when the ball's going to drop. (Boston Herald.)

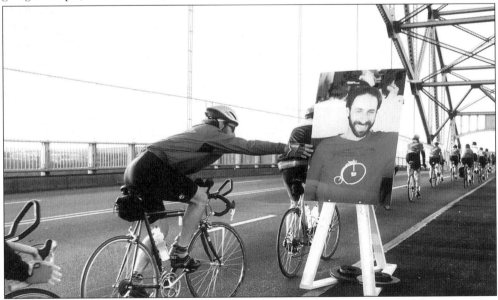

REMEMBERING TODD, 1998. The Pan-Massachusetts Challenge (PMC) bike-a-thon has always been an event deeply touched by emotion. The poster these cyclists are gently touching as they cross the Bourne Bridge during the 1998 ride is of Todd Miller, a longtime PMC supporter who lost his battle with cancer that spring. (Mark Turney photograph.)

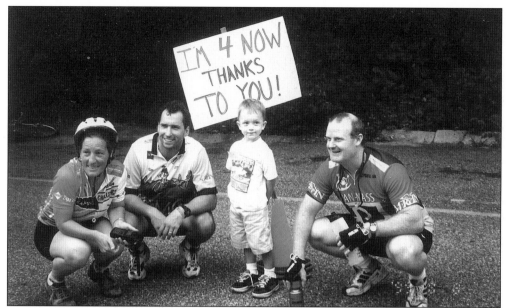

GIVING THANKS, 1999. Each year during the Pan-Massachusetts Challenge, riders look to little Jack O'Riordan and his hand-made signs for inspiration. Diagnosed with a rare cancer known as Wilms' tumor at age one, O'Riordan cheers participants annually at Nickerson State Park on Cape Cod. His 2000 sign read, "I'm 5 and Alive, Thanks to You." In 2001, the message changed to "I get to be 6, thanks to you." (Debra Ruder photograph.)

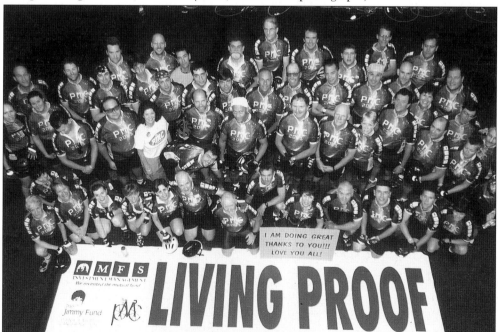

LIVING PROOF, 2001. The gathering of cancer survivors riding in the Pan-Massachusetts Challenge (PMC) is a highlight of each year's event. The 2001 PMC cycling contingent included 160 survivors; another 100 served during the weekend as volunteers. (Karen Cummings photograph.)

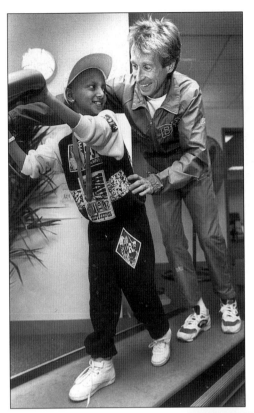

"BOSTON BILLY" RODGERS OFFERS TRAINING TIPS, SEPTEMBER 26, 1990. Since its inception in 1989, the Boston Marathon Jimmy Fund Walk has become one of Dana-Farber's most popular and profitable events. In this photograph, a guy who knows a little something about the famous 26.2-mile course—four-time Boston Marathon champion Bill Rodgers—helps Rena Parab of the Jimmy Fund Clinic get ready for the 1990 walk. (Boston Herald.)

HEROES HELP PASS THE MILES, C. THE 1990S. During each year's Jimmy Fund Walk, countless participants tap mile-markers featuring blown-up photographs of Jimmy Fund Clinic patient heroes along the route. Each image notes the patient's first name and career aspirations, as well as his or her own hero. (Steve Gilbert photograph.)

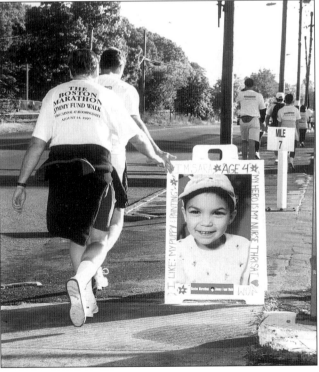

AN ADDED MESSAGE, SEPTEMBER 30, 2001. Each participant in the Jimmy Fund Walk receives a shirt emblazoned with that year's logo to wear during the event, and many walkers feel compelled to add personal tributes, photographs of loved ones lost to cancer, or team names to the design. For this 2001 entrant, the message was simple. (Steve Gilbert photograph.)

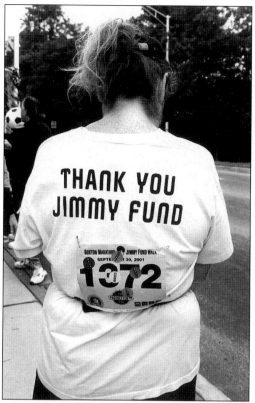

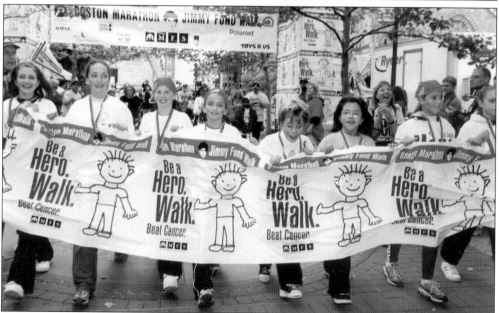

THE PATIENT-FAMILY CONTINGENT REACHES THE FINISH LINE, 2001. Nearly 8,500 people trekked all or part of the 26.2-mile route in the 2001 walk, none more inspiring than these Jimmy Fund Clinic patients and supporters shown proudly crossing the Copley Square finish line after their three-mile jaunt from the clinic. (Steve Gilbert photograph.)

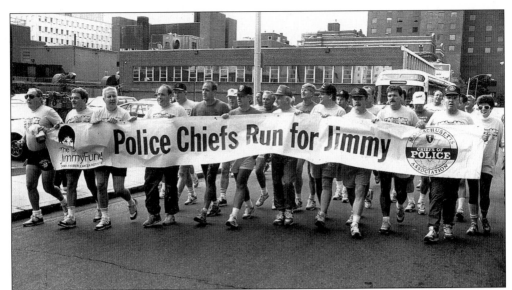

POLICE CHIEFS COMPLETE THE CROSS-COMMONWEALTH RUN, 1991. Each September, as a display of support for their official charity, members of the Massachusetts Chiefs of Police Association complete the "Chief Robert Mortell Run for Jimmy"—a 154-mile relay from the New York–Massachusetts border to Dana-Farber. There, they meet up with the patient-family contingent of the Jimmy Fund Walk and join it on the three-mile trip into Copley Square. (Boston Herald.)

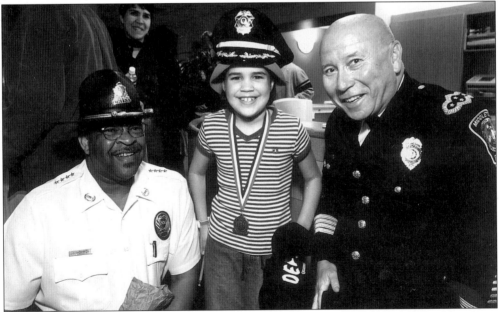

THE GOODWILL PATROL, 2000. In addition to their running exploits, the chiefs have been supporting the Jimmy Fund statewide through softball tournaments, picnics, and other means for a half-century. Nearly 50 chiefs make the association's annual Jimmy Fund Clinic visit, where they distribute badges to the young citizens on hand. Here, Barbara Barbosa dons Middleton Chief Paul Armitage's (right) hat while Chief James Thompson of Barre looks on. (Steve Gilbert photograph.)

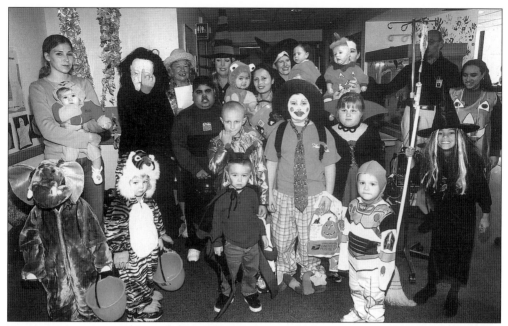

HALLOWEEN AT THE JIMMY FUND CLINIC, 2001. After each year's Jimmy Fund Walk, the next big event on the calendar for Dana-Farber's young patients is Halloween. Kids and their caregivers all dress up for the occasion, which includes trick-or-treating, a pizza party, and a staff pumpkin-carving contest. (Laura Wulf photograph.)

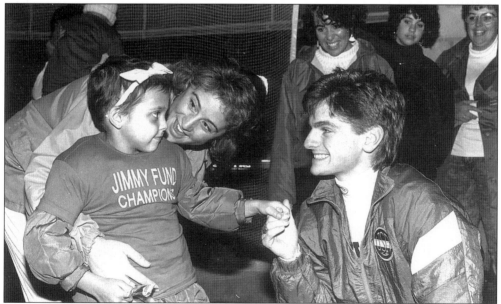

SILVER-MEDAL SMILES AT "AN EVENING WITH CHAMPIONS," THE EARLY 1990S. Since its 1970 inception, "An Evening with Champions" has grown into one of the Jimmy Fund's most unique and memorable late-autumn events. Spearheaded by volunteer efforts by students from Harvard College's Eliot House, the figure-skating fundraiser annually attracts some of the world's greatest performers—including 1992 Olympic Silver medalist and longtime event host Paul Wylie (right). (Steve Gilbert photograph.)

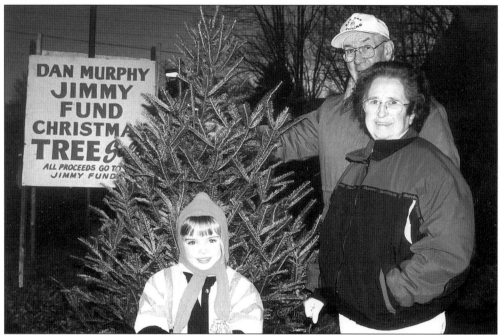

CHRISTMAS TREES FOR JIMMY, THE 1990S. If it's December, it's time for the Dan Murphy Jimmy Fund Christmas Tree Sale. For more than 30 years since their son Dan Murphy III was treated at Dana-Farber as a six-year-old, Dan Murphy Jr. and his wife, Priscilla, have been selling trees out of their Randolph, Massachusetts backyard, with all proceeds going to the Jimmy Fund. For their decades of dedication, the Murphys (shown with granddaughter Meagan Roach) were awarded the Yawkey Award. (Karen Cummings photograph.)

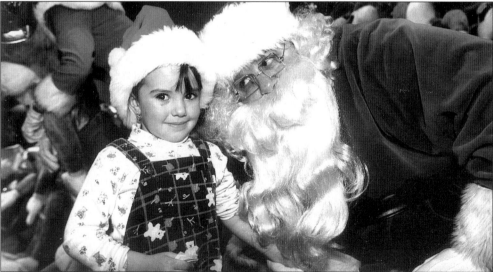

A JIMMY FUND CLINIC HOLIDAY PARTY, 1999. Also highlighting December is the annual Jimmy Fund Clinic holiday party, held off-campus. This Santa normally wears a stethoscope; he is Holcombe Grier, M.D., associate chief of Pediatric Oncology at DFCI. For close to 20 years, he has donned the red suit for photographs with clinic families, ably aided by medical fellows serving as elves. (Steve Gilbert photograph.)

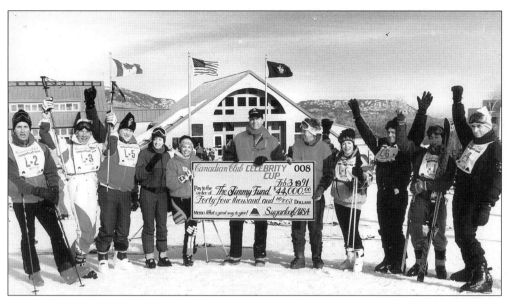

THE CANADIAN CLUB CELEBRITY CUP, 1991. Jimmy Fund ski events have long been a staple of the winter months. Held for more than 15 years starting in 1984, the Canadian Club Celebrity Cup at Sugarloaf offered participants three days of accommodations, entertainment, lift tickets, equipment, and the chance to ski with celebrities—including actor James Sikking (far right) and Olympic skier Diana Golden (holding left side of check) at the 1991 event. (Jimmy Fund.)

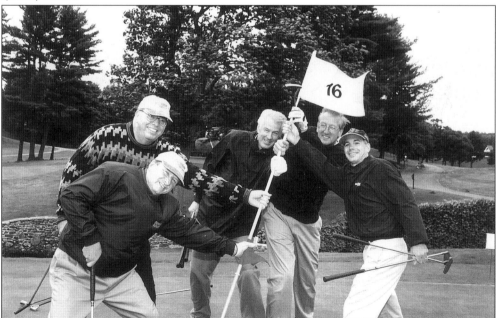

TEEING IT UP AT THE JIMMY FUND POLAROID GOLF CLASSIC, 1999. Starting each winter and going through October, the Jimmy Fund Golf Program offers more than 150 tournament opportunities to hit the links and help the cause. First officially run in 1982, the program now has venues from Maine to Florida and has raised more than $25 million for cancer research and treatment at Dana-Farber. (Steve Gilbert photograph.)

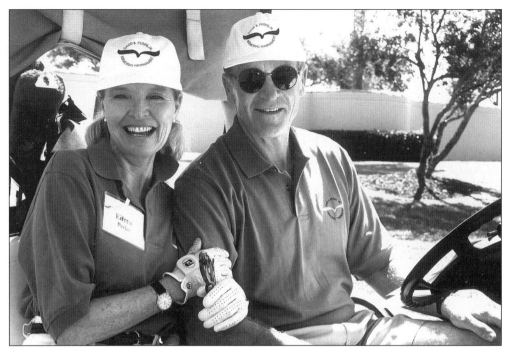

EILEEN AND DAVID PERINI SR. GOLFING FOR THEIR SON, 1999. The David B. Perini Jr. Memorial Golf Tournament, started in 1991, honors the life of its namesake—a patient at Dana-Farber and grandson of Jimmy Fund co-founder Louis Perini. All proceeds benefit the David B. Perini Jr. Quality of Life Clinic at DFCI, a multidisciplinary program founded by David's parents to provide care for survivors of childhood cancers and conduct research to better understand the long-term effects of pediatric cancer treatment. (Jimmy Fund.)

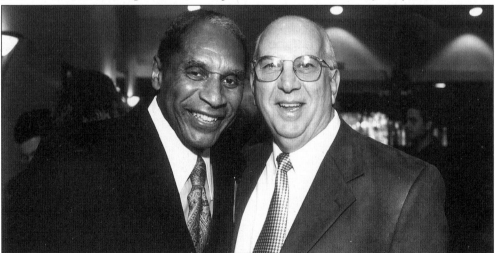

RON BURTON AND FRED DIGREGORIO AT THE JIMMY FUND GOLF CLASSIC, 2000. The Jimmy Fund Polaroid Golf Classic, held each fall, is a year-end tournament celebrating the growing success of the program. In this photograph, golf program director Fred DiGregorio (right) shares a moment with former Boston Patriots football player Ron Burton, a Dana-Farber supporter and patient who received the charity's annual Jimmy Award for his decades of giving. (Steve Gilbert photograph.)

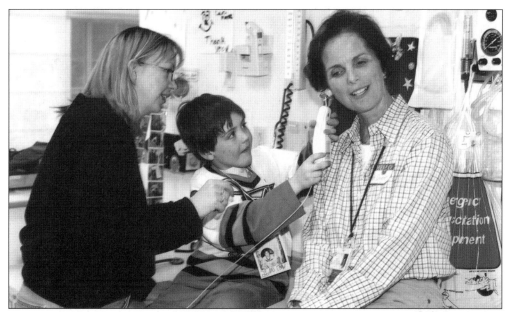

SIBLINGS TAKE THEIR TURN, APRIL 2001. Watching someone you love go through cancer treatment can be a frightening experience; to alleviate some of those concerns, Dana-Farber has held annual Sibling Days since 1986 for young brothers and sisters of Jimmy Fund Clinic patients to learn more about treatment. Here, Eorna Maguire (left) and Ian MacLean (center) give Patricia Dwyer, LICSW, of the clinic a "checkup." (Laura Wulf photograph.)

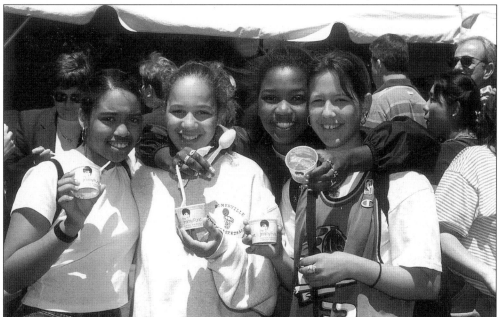

STICKY SMILES AT THE FLEET SCOOPER BOWL, JUNE 1999. As the weather starts to heat up each June, the Jimmy Fund offers a great way to cool off—the Fleet Scooper Bowl. The nation's largest all-you-can-eat ice-cream event, this annual three-day festival raised $110,000 for Dana-Farber in 2001 as some 35,000 gobblers of all ages consumed two million scoops of ice cream, frozen yogurt, and sorbet from nine sponsoring companies. (Gina Iannacchero photograph.)

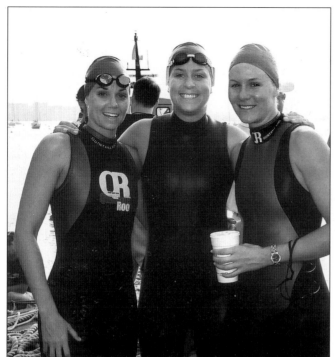

OLYMPIANS MAKE WAVES FOR DANA-FARBER, 2001. Summer gives water lovers the chance to crawl for cancer as part of the national Swim Across America program. Two Boston-area swims—one in Boston Harbor and one at Nantasket Beach—raise money to benefit Dana-Farber's David B. Perini Jr. Quality of Life Clinic and feature both elite and everyday participants. These U.S. Olympic medalists at the 2001 event are, from left to right, Ashley Tappen, Janel Jorgenson, and Jenny Thompson. (Janet Haley photograph.)

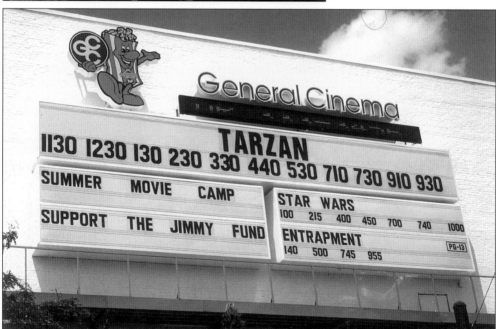

STILL MAKING MOVIE MAGIC, 1999. As the longest-running Jimmy Fund event (since 1949), the Jimmy Fund/Variety Club Theatre Collections Program continues to make summers a little more special for moviegoers. The Jimmy Fund trailer films shown before the feature presentations at more than 200 participating theaters remain immensely popular, and the collection canisters keep filling to record levels. Summer blockbusters, such as the *Star Wars* film on this marquee, always help. (Karen Cummings photograph.)

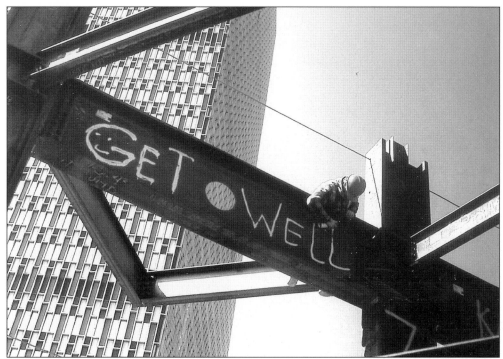

STRONG AS IRON, 2001. Inspired by a true story, the 2001 Jimmy Fund *Strong as Iron* film trailer moved moviegoers from Maine to Florida and garnered numerous awards. It tells the tale of the special bond created in 1996 between the ironworkers erecting the Richard A. and Susan F. Smith Research Laboratories on the Dana-Farber campus and the young cancer patients who watched them from the Jimmy Fund Clinic windows across the street. The two groups communicated through signs and spray paint, and the ironworkers began "passing the hard hat" for weekly donations to Dana-Farber. For the official premiere of the trailer, members of the Boston Iron Workers Union Local 7 who did the original construction and clinic patients from 1996 and beyond gathered to watch together. (Jimmy Fund.)

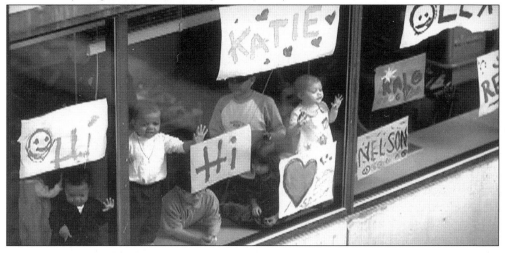

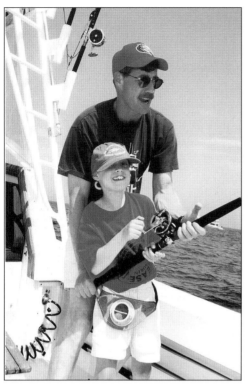

JOE CRONIN TOURNEY REELS IN FISH AND FUNDS, 2000. Jimmy Fund Clinic patient Chapin Moshen, eight, and his father, Tony, joined more than 200 anglers in the waters off Cape Cod for the seventh edition of the Joe Cronin Memorial Fishing Tournament in 2000. Honoring the late Red Sox shortstop and manager who was a longtime Jimmy Fund supporter, this annual August event hooked nearly $150,000 the following year. (Karen Cummings photograph.)

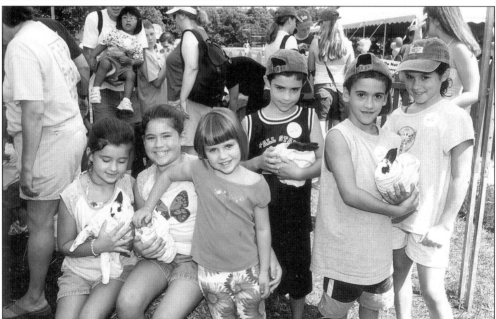

THE SUMMER FESTIVAL SHINES, 2001. Each summer since 1994, the Jimmy Fund Clinic summer festival has given patients past and present a day of fun in the sun with friends, family, and caregivers. Featuring pony rides, face painting, swimming, and more, the 2001 festival drew a record crowd of 1,400—including 300 patients. Here, some of the revelers have a hopping good time at the petting zoo. (Steve Gilbert photograph.)

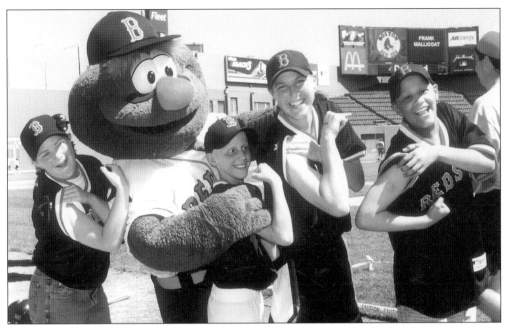

FANTASY DAY HITS A HOME RUN. Kids of all ages dream of stepping to the plate at Fenway Park and crushing a ball off its Green Monster left-field wall. The Jimmy Fund makes these dreams a reality through John Hancock Fantasy Day at Fenway. For a substantial gift to the Jimmy Fund, would-be sluggers get 15 chances to hit off a pitching machine at the hallowed ballpark; they also get their names read over the public address system and up in lights on the jumbo center-field scoreboard. Sponsor John Hancock makes additional contributions to the charity for every ball hit off or over the wall by adults and for all hits by Jimmy Fund Clinic patients that reach the outfield. The clinic quartet above muscled its way to $1,600 at the 2000 event to impress Wally the Green Monster. They are, from left to right, Lindsay Roache, Patrick White, Brendan Smith, and Stephen Fringuelli. (Steve Gilbert photographs.)

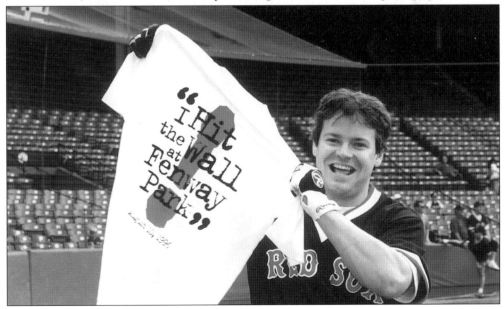

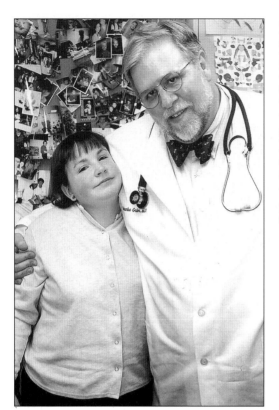

KATIE O'KEEFE AND DR. HOLCOMBE GRIER, 18-YEAR PARTNERS, 2001. Diagnosed with acute lymphoblastic leukemia at age four, Katie O'Keefe has suffered several challenges in the nearly two decades since her initial treatment in the Jimmy Fund Clinic. Helped each step of the way by her doctor of 18 years, Holcombe Grier, M.D., she now makes annual trips to the David B. Perini Jr. Quality of Life Clinic at Dana-Farber, which provides medical, education, and psychological services to childhood cancer survivors. (Laura Wulf photograph.)

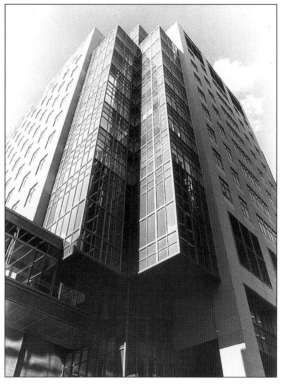

THE SMITH RESEARCH LABORATORIES OPEN, 1997. Dana-Farber's campus grew again with the completion in 1997 of the Richard A. and Susan F. Smith Research Laboratories. Endowed by its namesakes, both DFCI trustees, the 12-story structure provides space for more than 500 institute investigators, state-of-the-art laboratories, and an expanded library. (Steve Gilbert photograph.)

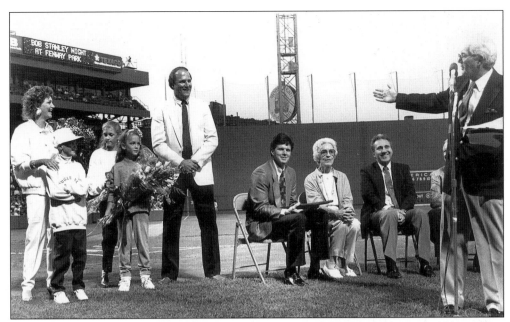

BOB STANLEY NIGHT AT FENWAY PARK, 1990. Few Red Sox players or spouses have been better friends to the Jimmy Fund through the years than longtime pitcher Bob Stanley and his wife, Joan. The couple's devotion to young patients took on added meaning when their own nine-year-old son, Kyle, was diagnosed with cancer and treated in the Jimmy Fund Clinic. In 1990—with their three children, including Kyle (in white cap), by their side—the Stanleys were honored with the Thomas A. Yawkey Award for their dedication. (Steve Gilbert photograph.)

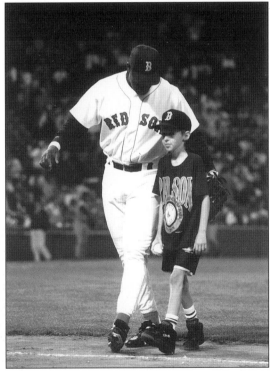

MO VAUGHN AND JASON LEADER, 1994. Slugger Mo Vaughn was another favorite of Jimmy Fund Clinic kids during his Red Sox career, and 11-year-old Jason Leader was no exception. When Vaughn called the young patient from California one night in April 1994 and said he would try to hit a homer for him and then delivered, an instant bond was formed. During a game at Fenway Park a few weeks later (right), Vaughn helped Leader throw out the first pitch. (Steve Gilbert photograph.)

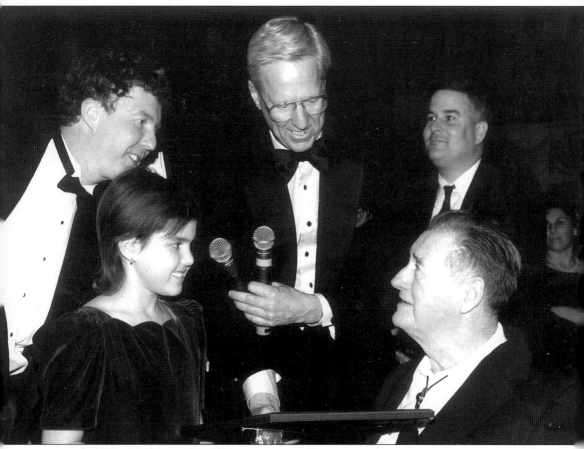

KATE SHAUGHNESSY AND TED WILLIAMS, DECEMBER 15, 1995. When Ted Williams (seated at right) was honored by the Jimmy Fund in 1995 as part of ceremonies to inaugurate the Ted Williams 406 Club at Dana-Farber, a special guest at the Park Plaza event was young Kate Shaughnessy. A Jimmy Fund Clinic patient who had received an encouraging phone call from Williams during her leukemia treatment through her father, *Boston Globe* sports columnist Dan Shaughnessy (left), Kate wrote a poem for Williams that she read to the crowd. (Steve Gilbert photograph.)

Ted Williams is a really, really great guy.
He really likes kids, but hates wearing ties.
He won two Triple Crowns, and was the MVP twice.
He feuded with sportswriters, but to kids he was nice.
521 homers, he's in the Hall of Fame,
He's the Kid, the Thumper, and Teddy Ballgame.
He would do anything for the Jimmy Fund,
And I'd like to say thank you, for all that he's done.

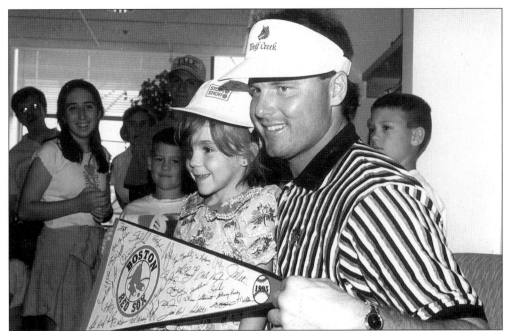

"ROCKET" ROGER CLEMENS PROVIDES A BOOST, 1995. Although this appearance in the Jimmy Fund Clinic was made on an off-afternoon, former Red Sox pitcher Roger Clemens was rumored to have occasionally made the short jog over to the clinic from Fenway Park for a quick hello on days he was slated to start. (Jimmy Fund.)

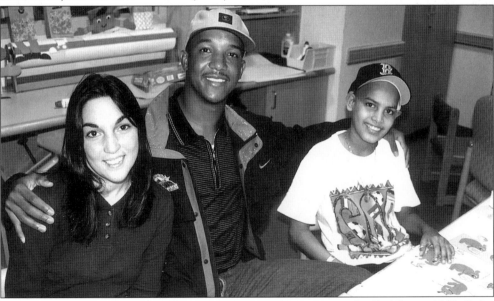

PEDRO MARTINEZ, JIMMY FUND CLINIC ACE, 1999. Since joining the Red Sox in 1998, Pedro Martinez has been a source of great support to the Jimmy Fund in two very different ways. The ace pitcher's visits have delighted young patients like these, and his massive strikeout totals have meant big contributions through the Hyundai Strike Out Cancer Campaign, in which the auto maker awards $50 to the charity for every whiff recorded by Red Sox hurlers. (Karen Cummings photograph.)

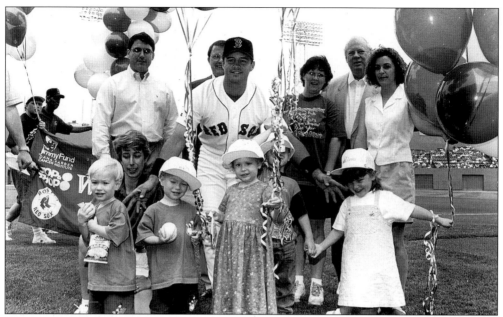

THE TRIPLE WINNER PROGRAM IS A HIT, THE 1990S. The Jimmy Fund's most successful corporate fundraiser in recent years has been the Stop & Shop Triple Winner Program, co-sponsored by the Red Sox. Jimmy Fund Clinic patients annually help promote and celebrate the program's success, as they did here at Fenway with help from former Sox infielder John Valentin (in uniform) and Stop & Shop CEO Marc Smith (far left). (Steve Gilbert photograph.)

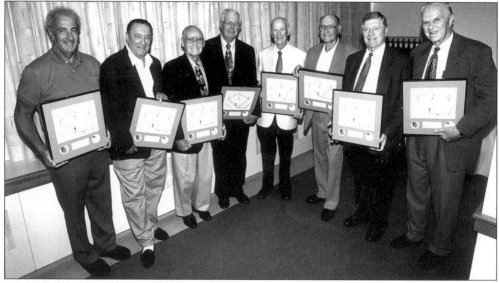

JIMMY'S BRAVES RETURN AFTER 49 YEARS, 1997. Labor Day weekend in 1997 brought a special group of visitors to Dana-Farber—players and staff from the original Boston Braves team that helped found the Jimmy Fund in 1948. The group toured the institute's research facilities and met kids in the Jimmy Fund Clinic. They are, from left to right, Charlie Chronopolus, Johnny Logan, Tommy Holmes, Art Johnson, Billy Sullivan, Sibby Sisti, Joe Morgan, and Johnny Sain. All were members of the Boston Braves Historical Association, which keeps alive memories of the team and the Jimmy Fund's formation. (Steve Gilbert photograph.)

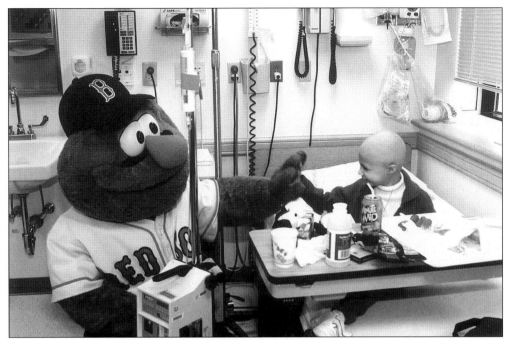

A HIGH-FIVE FROM WALLY, 1997. Red Sox appearances at the Jimmy Fund Clinic in recent years have not been limited to playing personnel. Team mascot Wally the Green Monster has also been a frequent guest, including one memorable trip in 1999 to pick up a "Good Luck" banner made by clinic patients to aid the team in its American League Championship Series against the dreaded Yankees. (Jimmy Fund.)

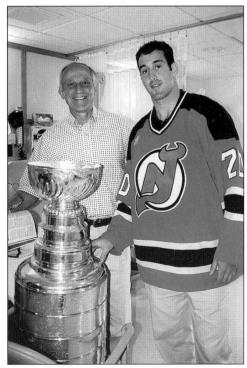

RAY PANDOLFO BRINGS THE STANLEY CUP TO DANA-FARBER, 2000. Jimmy Fund Clinic kids are not the only ones who enjoy the frequent celebrity visits at Dana-Farber. Here, an adult patent (left) shares a moment with Burlington, Massachusetts native Jay Pandolfo of the New Jersey Devils.

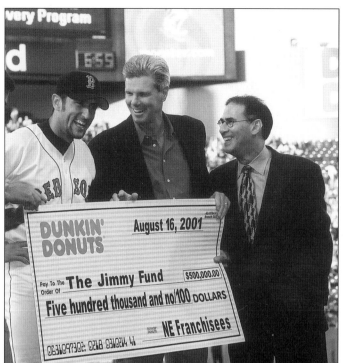

ANOTHER GIFT FOR THE JIMMY FUND, 2001. Since the days when Bill Koster was getting the Jimmy Fund off the ground, staff have been picking up oversized checks for the charity at assorted events. Here, Jimmy Fund chairman Mike Andrews (center) and Dr. Lee Nadler (right), vice president for Experimental Medicine at Dana-Farber, accept a gift from corporate sponsor Dunkin' Donuts at Fenway Park with help from Red Sox shortstop Nomar Garciaparra. (Steve Gilbert photograph.)

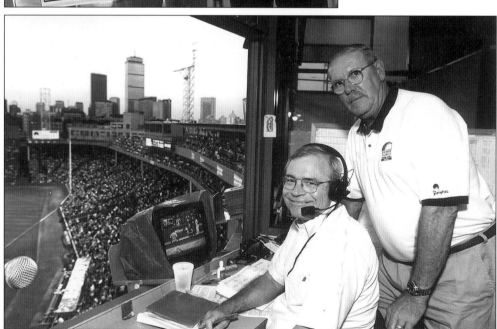

JOE CASTIGLIONE, VOICE OF THE RED SOX—AND THE JIMMY FUND, 1999. Like Ken Coleman, Curt Gowdy, and Jim Britt, Red Sox radio broadcaster Joe Castiglione (seated) has spent considerable time promoting the Jimmy Fund over the airwaves and volunteering as a toastmaster for the charity. In this photograph, Castiglione has yet another visitor in his booth to talk up the Jimmy Fund—Dunkin' Donuts franchise owner John Henderson. (Steve Gilbert photograph.)

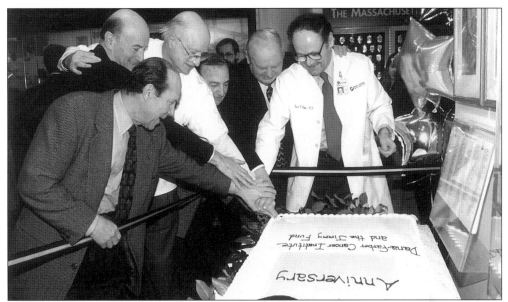

DANA-FARBER CELEBRATES ITS 50TH ANNIVERSARY, 1997. To mark a half-century since the founding of the Children's Cancer Research Foundation, Dana-Farber held a series of observances during 1997. The photograph above shows a January party held for staff and friends in the Dana building. The distinguished group cutting the cake includes, from left to right, DFCI trustees David Auerbach and Richard Morse; DFCI physician-in-chief emeritus Emil Frei III, M.D.; president emeritus Baruj Benacerraf, M.D.; former Boston Red Sox general manager Lou Gorman; and president David G. Nathan, M.D. In a separate ceremony, Deaconess Road (located between the Smith and Dana buildings) was renamed Jimmy Fund Way, as shown below. From left to right are Red Sox president John Harrington, Dr. David Nathan, and Carl Yastrzemski. (Steve Gilbert photographs.)

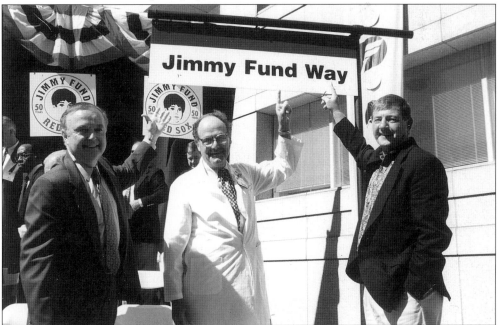

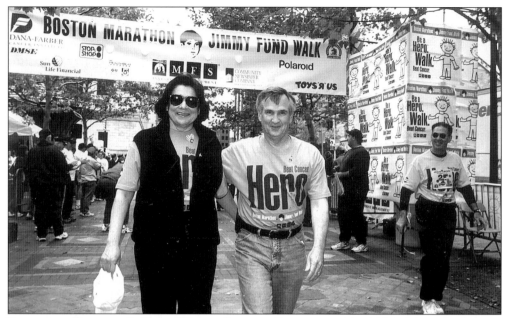

PRESIDENT EDWARD J. BENZ WALKS PROUD, SEPTEMBER 30, 2001. Many fundraising organizations canceled events in the days following the terrorist attacks of September 11, 2001, but Dana-Farber president Edward J. Benz Jr., M.D., and event organizers felt the Jimmy Fund Walk should go on. Amid a patriotic display of red, white, and blue, some 8,500 people put aside fears and pounded the pavement—including Benz and his wife, Margaret Vettese, Ph.D., R.N., seen here crossing the finish line. (Steve Gilbert photograph.)

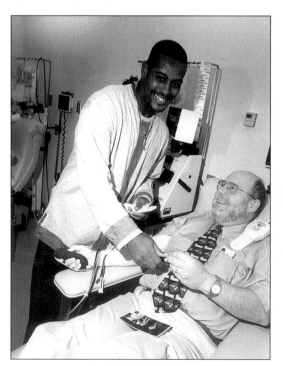

PATRIOTS HELP DANA-FARBER PROMOTE PLATELET DONATIONS, FALL 2001. Nearly 20 years after his family first endowed Dana-Farber's blood donor facility, New England Patriots owner and Dana-Farber trustee Robert Kraft encouraged his football team to help promote public donations of platelets—life-saving clotting agents in blood. Here, Patriots star cornerback Ty Law (left) does his part by visiting with platelet donor David Smith in the Kraft Family Blood Donor Center. (Eric Antoniou photograph.)

THE JIMMY FUND WEB SITE, 2002. To provide detailed information about its events, programs, and new opportunities for volunteering or making gifts, the Jimmy Fund launched a revamped Web site in 2001, www.jimmyfund.org. The site links to the latest DFCI tips for finding a doctor and even lets users view old Jimmy Fund movie trailers or listen to the original Jimmy radio broadcast. (Jimmy Fund.)

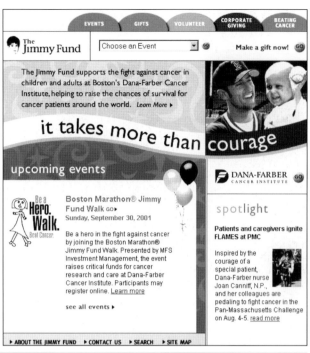

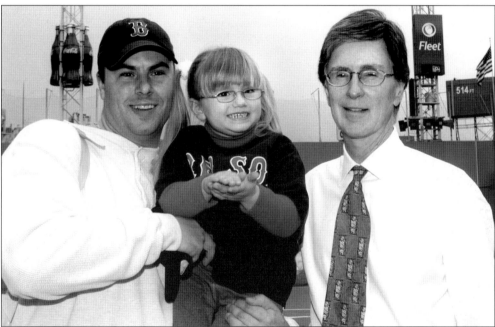

NEW RED SOX OWNERS SUSTAIN THE JIMMY FUND RELATIONSHIP, 2002. When the new Boston Red Sox ownership group led by John Henry, Tom Werner, and Larry Lucchino took control of the club in early 2002, it quickly announced the team would maintain the Jimmy Fund as its official charity. Special plans to mark the 50th anniversary of the relationship were planned, and Henry (right) quickly got acquainted with VIPs like Gabby Lukas (center), Jimmy Fund spokespatient for the Stop & Shop Triple Winner Program, and her father, Jeff. (Steve Gilbert photograph.)

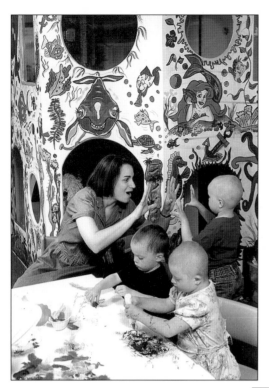

"THE PLAY LADY" AT WORK, THE LATE 1990S. Her name is Lisa Scherber, but around the Jimmy Fund Clinic, everybody knows her as "the Play Lady." Activities coordinator for the clinic since the early 1990s, Scherber keeps patients and their families happy during visits by knowing just which toy, video, treat, or reassuring comment they need. She also supervises the clinic's corps of volunteers and organizes its many successful outreach programs. (Josh Touster photograph.)

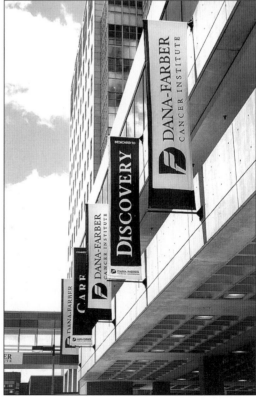

DEDICATED TO DISCOVERY . . . COMMITTED TO CARE. The message on these two banners outside the Dana building is also the official slogan for Dana-Farber Cancer Institute. It embodies the dual goals that have guided Dana-Farber and the Jimmy Fund since 1948—seeking tomorrow's cancer cures while providing the best possible treatment for today's patients. (Jimmy Fund.)

116

Six

JIMMY AND TED RETURN: 1998–2001

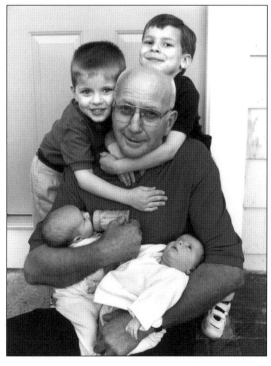

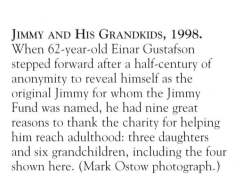

JIMMY AND HIS GRANDKIDS, 1998.
When 62-year-old Einar Gustafson
stepped forward after a half-century of
anonymity to reveal himself as the
original Jimmy for whom the Jimmy
Fund was named, he had nine great
reasons to thank the charity for helping
him reach adulthood: three daughters
and six grandchildren, including the four
shown here. (Mark Ostow photograph.)

For the first half-century of the Jimmy Fund's existence, almost everybody connected with the charity felt certain of one thing: the original Jimmy for whom it was named had not survived his 1948 bout with cancer. Very few children diagnosed in that era recovered, and although several individuals had claimed over the decades to be the 12-year-old boy whose poignant radio interview had launched nationwide support for Dr. Sidney Farber's research, none had proven the real deal. Jimmy represented every child with cancer, but he was surely gone.

Then, just as the 50th anniversary of its founding approached, an event occurred very much in keeping with the Hollywood-like beginnings of the Jimmy Fund. Before heading off on vacation, Jimmy Fund chairman Mike Andrews handed Karen Cummings, assistant director of Communications at Dana-Farber, a letter from a woman claiming her brother was Jimmy. Andrews had seen similar letters prove unworthy but had a feeling this one might be different. When Cummings read the woman's remembrances of sitting by the radio and hearing her brother sing "Take Me Out to the Ballgame" during his 1948 interview, she felt compelled to pursue the lead. A short while later, she received the following message on her answering machine: "Hello, Karen? This is Jimmy. Heard you were looking for me."

It was Einar "Jimmy" Gustafson—alive and well and living a quiet life in northern Maine as a 62-year-old truck driver and grandfather of six. Gustafson's story checked out with medical records still on file at Children's Hospital Boston, and when Cummings met him for the first time in a Chelsea, Massachusetts parking lot in early March, she got the clincher. Playing a cassette tape of the original Ralph Edwards broadcast for Gustafson over her car radio, she saw tears well up in his eyes.

It was a case of perfect timing. Gustafson was given a hero's welcome at Dana-Farber during the week of the charity's 50th anniversary, where staff and patients stood in line awaiting his autograph. On May 22, 50 years *to the day* of his radio broadcast, the Boston Red Sox invited him to throw out the first pitch at Fenway Park before a game with the Yankees. His reemergence prompted stories in *People, Sports Illustrated,* and newspapers across the country, and he filmed a public service announcement for Dana-Farber.

Asked why he had not stepped forward earlier, the soft-spoken, six-foot-three Gustafson said simply that he had considered it but was always too busy with his family and job. Friends and neighbors back in his tiny hometown of New Sweden knew, and they also kept quiet. He had even stayed in touch for decades with his doctor, Sidney Farber, who in several newspaper articles before his 1973 death stated that the original Jimmy was a healthy young man raising a family—a detail somehow lost over the years.

Yet once Gustafson's identity *was* revealed, he was anything but reticent. Despite a demanding job that often had him driving his truck throughout the country, he made countless volunteer appearances on behalf of Dana-Farber. He did everything from serve as grand marshal of the Boston Marathon Jimmy Fund Walk to transport bicycles to and from Cape Cod in his 18-wheeler during the Pan-Massachusetts Challenge bike-a-thon.

The high point of "Jimmy-mania" came in July 1999, when Gustafson met for the first time the man who spent a half-century raising awareness and countless dollars for the Jimmy Fund: Boston Red Sox legend Ted Williams. As the two embraced in the Jimmy Fund Clinic before a sea of young patients and news cameras, it was if the entire history of the charity had come full circle.

Sadly, Dana-Farber's time with Gustafson was all too brief. He died at age 65 on January 21, 2001, after suffering a stroke. In the end, he spent less than three years spreading the Jimmy Fund message, but by giving selflessly to the organization that had saved his life, he in turn gave hope to many others facing their own disease.

"Einar's story—that he was cured at a time when so few were and led such a full life—is an inspiration to all of us," DFCI president Edward J. Benz Jr., M.D., said upon Gustafson's death. "His story is the story of our nation's war on cancer, and over the past five decades, tens of thousands of people have rallied against cancer in his name. We certainly pledge to continue that fight."

KAREN CUMMINGS MEETS EINAR "JIMMY" GUSTAFSON, MARCH 1998. By the time Karen Cummings of Dana-Farber met Einar Gustafson in this Chelsea, Massachusetts parking lot, she was confident he was the original Jimmy. Final verification for her skeptical colleagues would come when she made the 417-mile drive to Gustafson's home and saw the original woolen Boston Braves uniform and bat given to him by the team in 1948. Back then, Gustafson had regularly made the same trek over two-lane roads to his checkups with Dr. Farber. (Gloria Gustafson photograph.)

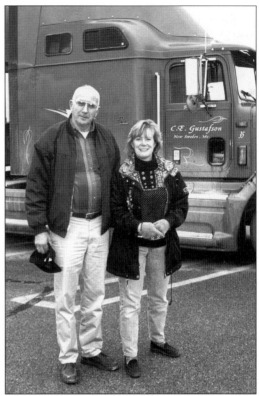

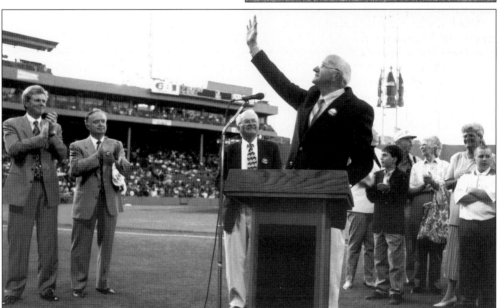

THE HALF-CENTURY SALUTE AT FENWAY PARK, MAY 22, 1998. Fifty years to the day of the original Jimmy broadcast, the Boston Red Sox honored Einar Gustafson with a ceremony at Fenway Park. The man who had launched the team's official charity as a 12-year-old cancer patient received a standing ovation from the crowd, which heard portions of the 1948 radio interview over the loudspeakers. (Jimmy Fund.)

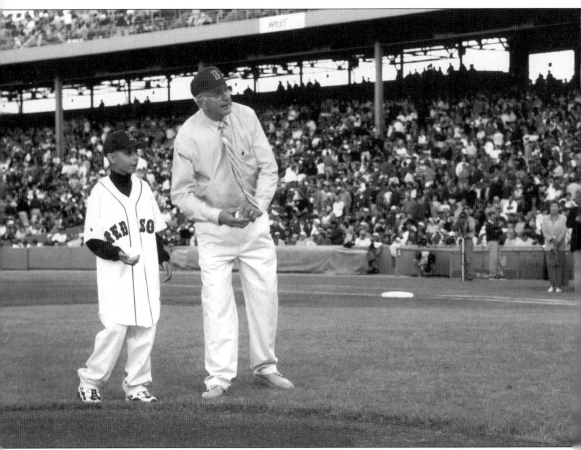

EINAR GUSTAFSON AND XAVIER "NEW JIMMY" LUGO SHARE FIRST-PITCH HONORS, MAY 22, 1998. When Einar Gustafson was invited to throw out the first pitch before the Red Sox–Yankees game that followed his May 22 salute at Fenway Park, he was joined by 11-year-old Xavier Lugo. A Jimmy Fund Clinic patient being treated for acute lymphoblastic leukemia (ALL)—the same disease for which Dr. Sidney Farber and his team of researchers were the first to attain temporary remissions back in 1947—Lugo symbolized the "new generation of Jimmys" now living with cancer. Like Gustafson a half-century before, he was presented with an authentic uniform jersey from his favorite team on the occasion. (Jimmy Fund.)

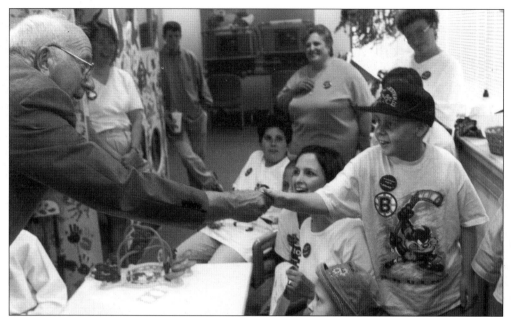

AN INSPIRATIONAL VISIT TO THE JIMMY FUND CLINIC, MAY 21, 1998. The day before his Fenway appearance, Gustafson enjoyed an emotional return to the Jimmy Fund Clinic. There, he met with young patients and their families, including one mother who told him how inspiring it was to see a grandfather who had once had the same disease for which her son was currently being treated. (Jimmy Fund.)

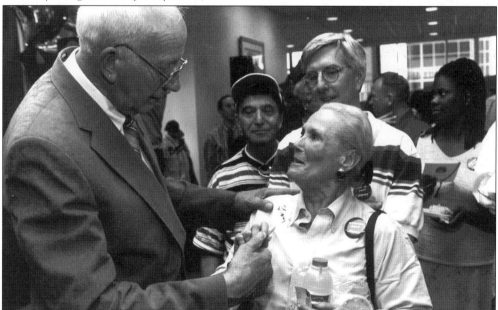

A HERO'S WELCOME, MAY 1998. After his clinic appearance, Gustafson met with Dana-Farber staff members, patients, and volunteers during a poignant welcome-back reception. People lined up for handshakes and autographs, and Gustafson patiently spoke to each one. Most fans had special event programs for him to sign, but longtime front-desk volunteer Fifi Swerling Kellem preferred having Jimmy inscribe her shirt. (Jimmy Fund.)

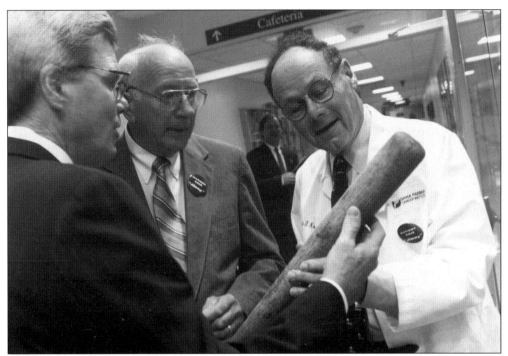

A Storied Bat, May 1998. Einar Gustafson (center) took a special tour of the Dana-Farber research facilities with institute president David G. Nathan, M.D., (right) and Jimmy Fund chairman Mike Andrews. Later, they examined the Earl Torgeson bat Gustafson had received from the Boston Braves first baseman five decades earlier. (Steve Gilbert photograph.)

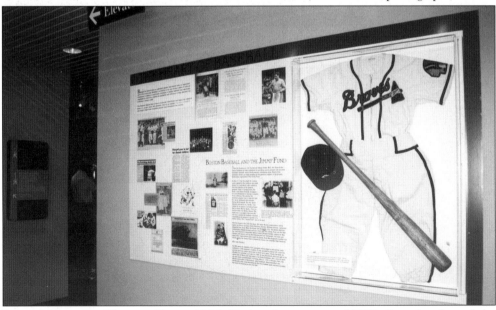

Jimmy Makes the Hall of Fame, 1998. During the summer of 1998, Gustafson loaned the Boston Braves uniform, bat, and cap he had received from his boyhood heroes in 1948 to the National Baseball Hall of Fame in Cooperstown, New York. There, they were displayed in a exhibit on the game and its community ties. (National Baseball Hall of Fame.)

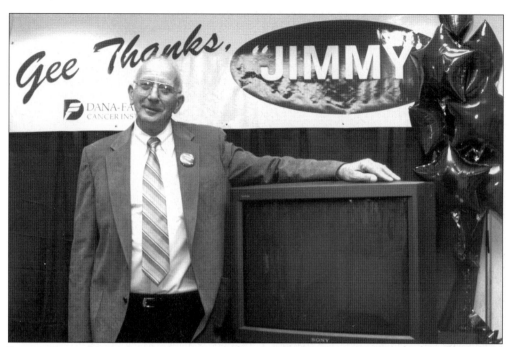

Jimmy Gets Another Television, 1998. In the tradition of the original 1948 radio broadcast (see page 20), Einar Gustafson was given a television set, courtesy of Sony, during the welcome-back ceremony held in his honor at Dana-Farber. (Jimmy Fund.)

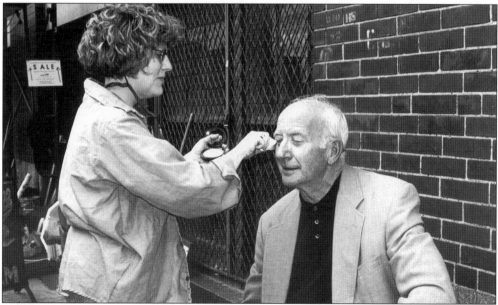

Spreading the Word of Hope, 1999. One thing Gustafson likely saw a few times on his new set was the Jimmy Fund public service announcement he recorded during 1999. In the spot, which aired on various Boston-area television stations in 1999 and 2000, footage of Gustafson walking the streets of Boston is interspersed with a simulation of his 1948 visits to Dana-Farber as a child. "My face used to stand for how long a child could live with cancer," he said in the announcement. "Now my face stands for how long a child can live *without* cancer." (Jimmy Fund.)

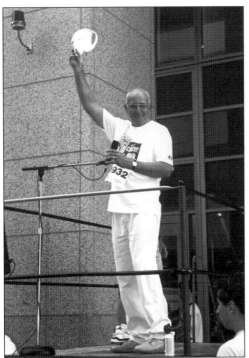

EINAR GUSTAFSON, JIMMY FUND WALK GRAND MARSHAL, 1998. Four months after his welcome home at Dana-Farber, Einar Gustafson served as grand marshal of the 1998 Boston Marathon Jimmy Fund Walk. Standing just a few hundred yards from the Jimmy Fund Clinic his story had helped build, he saluted participants in the three-mile Patient-Family Walk as they left Dana-Farber. (Jimmy Fund.)

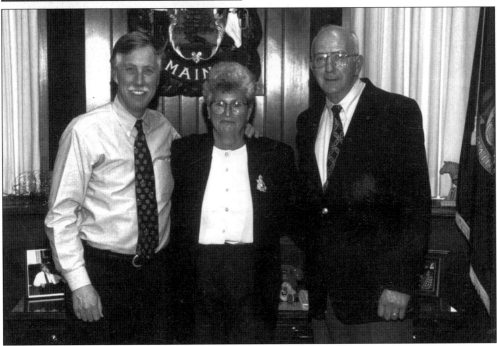

MAINE DECLARES JIMMY DAY AGAIN, APRIL 1999. When the Jimmy Fund was first formed in the summer of 1948, all six New England states had declared "Jimmy Days" in honor of an anonymous 12-year-old cancer patient. A half-century later, with the boy's identity revealed to be that of Maine native Einar Gustafson, Gov. Angus King (left) repeated the tribute for his state's favorite son (right) and Gustafson's wife, Gloria. (Jimmy Fund.)

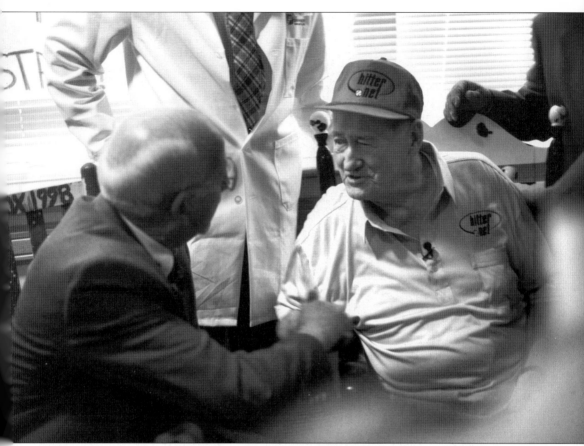

EINAR GUSTAFSON AND TED WILLIAMS—"HIYA, JIMMY BABY," JULY 1999. It seemed nothing could match the drama of Einar "Jimmy" Gustafson's first return to Dana-Farber in 50 years, but the initial meeting between Gustafson (left) and Red Sox legend Ted Williams on July 9, 1999, was every bit as powerful. The two men whose names are synonymous with the Jimmy Fund came together in the most appropriate of locales—a Jimmy Fund Clinic playroom filled with laughing young patients. It was an especially dramatic moment for the 80-year-old Williams, who had spent a half-century helping raise countless dollars for the Jimmy Fund as its "All-Time All Star." "Hiya, Jimmy baby!" he yelled, a wide grin crossing his face, "Boy, you look great! How'd you get so big?" (Jimmy Fund.)

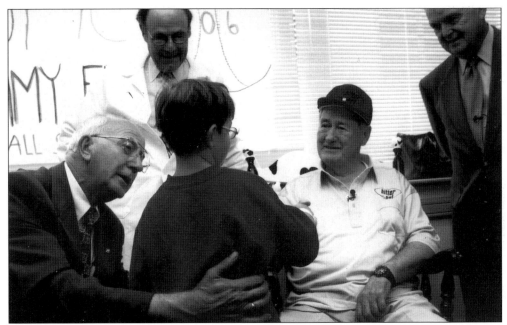

A GENTLE HAND, JULY 1999. After Einar Gustafson (left) and Ted Williams (seated) first met up in the Jimmy Fund Clinic, they sat and talked with a long line of young patients and family members. Joining them in this view are Dana-Farber president David G. Nathan, M.D., (in white coat) and Boston Red Sox president John Harrington, also a Dana-Farber trustee. (Jimmy Fund.)

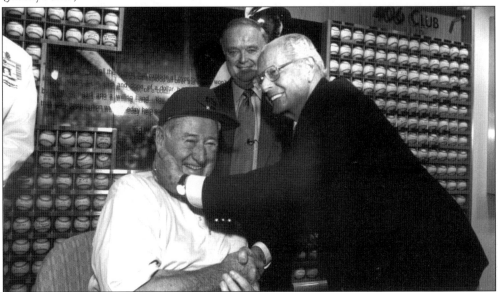

TED WILLIAMS AND DOM DIMAGGIO AT DANA-FARBER, JULY 1999. Next up for Williams after his visit with Gustafson was a trip downstairs to the Ted Williams Jimmy Fund Gallery, a series of display cases named in his honor and featuring a timeline history of the charity and Dana-Farber. There, he caught up with former Red Sox teammate and fellow Dana-Farber trustee Dom DiMaggio (right) in front of a display devoted to the Ted Williams 406 Club as John Harrington looked on behind them. (Steve Gilbert photograph.)

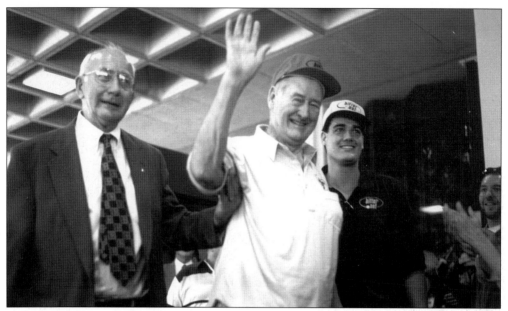

TED AND JIMMY SAY GOODBYE, JULY 1999. An admiring crowd gathered outside the Dana building when Einar "Jimmy" Gustafson and Ted Williams emerged at the end of their July 1999 visit. After walking by the cheering throngs with Williams' son John Henry (right), the two Jimmy Fund icons embraced before Williams stepped into a car and drove off past the Jimmy Fund Building. It was to be their only meeting. (Jimmy Fund.)

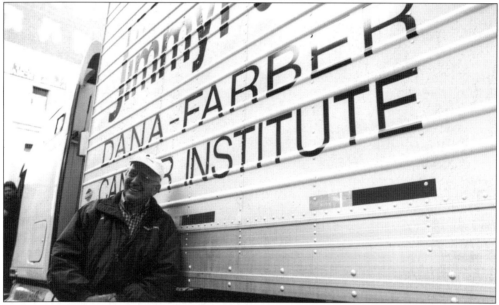

JIMMY AND DANA-FARBER HIT THE HIGHWAYS, DECEMBER 1999. In a special ceremony on Jimmy Fund Way, Chancellor Corporation, a Boston-based leasing company and Dana-Farber sponsor, surprised Gustafson with an early Christmas present of a new refrigerator trailer for his truck in December 1999. The institute had the Jimmy Fund logo and tagline emblazoned on the side of the trailer, so Gustafson could take the message—"Because it takes more than courage to beat cancer"—nationwide. (Steve Gilbert photograph.)

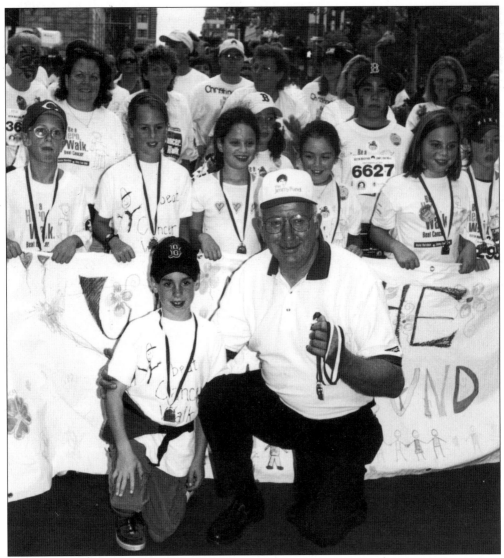

EINAR GUSTAFSON, THE PERFECT JIMMY. Just over three months after he presented medals to finishers at the 2000 Boston Marathon Jimmy Fund Walk (above), 65-year-old Einar Gustafson died on January 21, 2001, after suffering a stroke. His death, like that of Dr. Sidney Farber 28 years before, prompted an outpouring of emotion of the Dana-Farber campus. A memorial service was held for Gustafson in the Jimmy Fund Auditorium, and representatives from the institute, including Jimmy Fund chairman Mike Andrews and Dana-Farber president emeritus David G. Nathan, M.D., flew to northern Maine for his funeral. "If we had tried to create a grown-up 'Jimmy,' we couldn't have come up with a better man than the real one," Andrews said during this time. "He was absolutely genuine—a completely kind, gentle, and generous man." (Steve Gilbert photograph.)

"My favorite part of coming forward has been going to the Jimmy Fund Clinic and seeing the kids. The kids are so young, they don't think about what's happening to them or what made their treatments possible. They just want to go home, like I did."

—Einar "Jimmy" Gustafson